The Professional Nurse Advocate's Handbook

The Professional Nurse Advocate's Handbook

Edited by

Liz Lees-Deutsch

Emma Wadey

and

Rosie Kneafsey

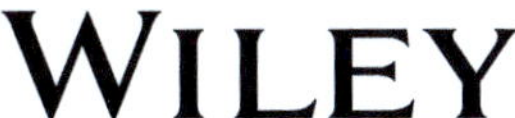

Registered Office(s)
John Wiley & Sons, Inc., 111 River Street, Hoboken, NJ 07030, USA
John Wiley & Sons Ltd, New Era House, 8 Oldlands Way, Bognor Regis, West Sussex, PO22 9NQ, UK

For details of our global editorial offices, customer services, and more information about Wiley products visit us at www.wiley.com.

Wiley also publishes its books in a variety of electronic formats and by print-on-demand. Some content that appears in standard print versions of this book may not be available in other formats.

Limit of Liability/Disclaimer of Warranty
The contents of this work are intended to further general scientific research, understanding, and discussion only and are not intended and should not be relied upon as recommending or promoting scientific method, diagnosis, or treatment by physicians for any particular patient. In view of ongoing research, equipment modifications, changes in governmental regulations, and the constant flow of information relating to the use of medicines, equipment, and devices, the reader is urged to review and evaluate the information provided in the package insert or instructions for each medicine, equipment, or device for, among other things, any changes in the instructions or indication of usage and for added warnings and precautions. While the publisher and the authors have used their best efforts in preparing this work, including a review of the content of the work, neither the publisher nor the authors make any representations or warranties with respect to the accuracy or completeness of the contents of this work and specifically disclaim all warranties, including without limitation any implied warranties of merchantability or fitness for a particular purpose. No warranty may be created or extended by sales representatives, written sales materials or promotional statements for this work. The fact that an organization, website, or product is referred to in this work as a citation and/or potential source of further information does not mean that the publisher and authors endorse the information or services the organization, website, or product may provide or recommendations it may make. This work is sold with the understanding that the publisher is not engaged in rendering professional services. The advice and strategies contained herein may not be suitable for your situation. You should consult with a specialist where appropriate. Further, readers should be aware that websites listed in this work may have changed or disappeared between when this work was written and when it is read. Neither the publisher nor authors shall be liable for any loss of profit or any other commercial damages, including
but not limited to special, incidental, consequential, or other damages.

Library of Congress Cataloging-in-Publication Data
Names: Lees-Deutsch, Liz editor | Wadey, Emma editor | Kneafsey, Rosie
  editor
Title: The professional nurse advocate's handbook / edited by Liz
  Lees-Deutsch, Emma Wadey, and Rosie Kneafsey.
Description: First edition. | Hoboken, NJ: John Wiley & Sons, Inc, 2026. |
  Includes index.
Identifiers: LCCN 2026003443 (print) | LCCN 2026003444 (ebook) | ISBN
  9781394308071 paperback | ISBN 9781394308095 adobe pdf | ISBN
  9781394308088 epub
Subjects: LCSH: Nurse practitioners | Nurses–Training | LCGFT: Handbooks
  and manuals
Classification: LCC RT82.8 .P77 2026 (print) | LCC RT82.8 (ebook) | DDC
  610.7306/92–dc23/eng/20260317
LC record available at https://lccn.loc.gov/2026003443
LC ebook record available at https://lccn.loc.gov/2026003444

Cover Design: Wiley
Cover Image: © SEAN GLADWELL/Getty Images
Set in 10.5/13pt STIXTwoText by Straive, Pondicherry, India
Printed and bound by CPI Group (UK) Ltd, Croydon, CR0 4YY
C9781394308071_010626
The manufacturer's authorized representative according to the EU
General Product Safety Regulation is Wiley-VCH GmbH, Boschstr.
12, 69469 Weinheim, Germany, e-mail: Product_Safety@wiley.com.

Contents

About the Editors

Liz Lees-Deutsch

Liz Lees-Deutsch is a professor of nursing practice based in the Centre for Care Excellence, a collaborative partnership between Coventry University and University Hospitals Coventry and Warwickshire. Over her 35-year registered nursing career, she worked in both the United Kingdom and the United States. She has published over 150 academic papers on a broad range of topics to include patient discharge through qualitative enquiry, and acute medicine nursing, where she was a consultant nurse for 20 years. She has authored two multi-professional patient discharge textbooks and travelled globally to deliver invited lectures and conference presentations on practice-based topics. In 2016, she was awarded a life fellowship of the Society for Acute Medicine for her contributions to the development of nursing. In 2023, she took up her current clinical academic role. She led the national evaluation of PNA programmes in 2022 and 2025 to evaluate the PNA Programme (SUSTAIN) and the impact of PNAs on patient experiences through quality improvement (SUSTAIN-ING). This work is now being taken forward through a national quality improvement toolkit, with more work proposed.

Professor Emma Wadey

Professor Emma Wadey is the Deputy Chief Executive and Chief Nursing Officer at Hertfordshire Partnership University NHS Foundation Trust and was formerly the National Deputy Director for Mental Health Nursing at NHSE England. Enthusiastic about the provision and transformation of effective and recovery-based mental health services, she has led the development of new and innovative services for the most vulnerable in our society. During COVID, she was the clinical lead for the National Mental Health, response cell and technical advisor to WHO, providing expert clinical oversight during the pandemic. During her career, she has specialised in the prevention of suicide and promotion of health and well-being, for both communities and healthcare staff, including the development of national suicide prevention toolkits. She led the implementation of professional nurse advocates to all healthcare settings and worked with Liz and Rosie during the national evaluation.

Professor Rosie Kneafsey

Professor Rosie Kneafsey is an experienced educational leader, researcher and practitioner with a 25- year academic career. In her current role, she is the Academic Director for CU Health and Care (Coventry University), which provides under-graduate, post-graduate and apprenticeship education in nursing, midwifery and the allied health professions. Professor Kneafsey's research centres on workforce development and well-being and seeks to support the development of a sustainable healthcare workforce for the future, through effective training and education; support for resilience and mental health; and application effective leadership approaches within organisational contexts. Professor Kneafsey provides supervision to numerous PhD candidates, and enjoys supporting colleagues to secure opportunities for scholarship and personal growth.

Notes on Contributors

Dr Analisa Smythe

Analisa qualified as a mental health nurse in 1993 and has worked in research for over 20 years. She has a significant track record of grant funding and has written numerous papers for publication. She was appointed as Research Matron at the Royal Wolverhampton NHS Trust in 2020 – a bespoke role established to enhance the reputation of the Trust for nursing research and build capacity and capability across the workforce. She is also a nurse researcher at Birmingham and Solihull Mental Health Foundation Trust and a visiting fellow at the University of Staffordshire and Nottingham Trent University. Her current interests focus on roles which support the well-being of the nursing workforce including the professional nurse advocate role.

Clare Capito

Clare is a senior midwife and national leader in professional advocacy and supervision. Appointed in 2001 as one of England's first consultant midwives, she has led service and workforce improvements across London. She helped develop the A-EQUIP model from its inception and led its implementation in London, embedding the professional midwifery advocate (PMA) role. Since 2022, she has led the national PMA programme and, in 2023, became the first Head of the PMA programme for NHS England.

Originally a registered nurse (1983), Clare has also led the regional professional nurse advocate (PNA) programme for London since September 2021, supporting rollout across 37 trusts and developing a network of 1,008 PNAs. Working part-time across both the PMA and PNA programmes, she champions A-EQUIP as a practical model for strengthening staff wellbeing and improving the quality of care for women, babies and families.

In January 2026, Kingston University London awarded Clare an honorary Doctor of the University degree (honoris causa) in recognition of her outstanding contribution to midwifery.

Adele Parsons

Adele is an advanced clinical practitioner (ACP), senior lecturer and programme lead for the professional advocacy programmes at the University of Lincoln. With a background in nursing and advanced clinical practice, she brings extensive experience in supporting healthcare professionals through education, supervision and reflective practice. Her academic and professional focus lies in restorative clinical supervision and its potential to cultivate compassionate, resilient and connected healthcare teams. Guided by Maya Angelou's belief that *"people will forget what you said, people will forget what you did, but people will never forget how you made them feel,"* Adele works to strengthen cultures of care, emotional well-being and professional integrity. She is committed to promoting restorative approaches that protect colleagues from burnout and compassion fatigue, enhancing team cohesion and reflective capacity. It is her hope that the chapter on restorative clinical supervision provides both inspiration and practical insights to help teams care for themselves as they care for others.

Jill Barr

Jill Barr, a lecturer at Coventry University, supervises student nurses and MBA/MSc students in health care. She trained as a nurse, midwife and health visitor, gaining a number of academic qualifications and a Michigan nurse license abroad. She worked as a head of academic studies and a principal lecturer at the University of Wolverhampton and De Montfort University, overseeing awards from pre-registration and specialist community nursing, non-medical prescribing, physician assistant/associate, advanced practitioner and public health masters. This involved managing a wide range of partnerships between NHS Trusts and other parts of the wider UK health industry to support workforce plans and new roles. She has had a particular interest in leadership/management in health care for many years and co-published seven texts to support future leaders in health care and improve patient care and outcomes. The professional nurse advocate (PNA) role has been of particular interest to further quality improvement in the NHS.

Martin Hogan

Martin Hogan has been a registered adult nurse since 2008. Clinical background as a Macmillan specialist nurse in Acute Oncology, intensive care and cardiology. After the first wave of COVID, his career has been very different. Having worked for the RCN as a senior regional officer for Surrey to then working within Mental health as the lead for the postgraduate portfolio in education and workforce development, where she undertook his professional nurse advocate course, which led him to become the lead PNA and move in the community for a full-time lead PNA role four days a week within the NHS. He has graduated as a QI coach, Florence Nightingale scholar and executive coach at Cambridge University. Recently, he has set up a not-for-profit company called the Improvement Coalition, where he is the co-director for organisational development and consultancy.

Bethany Hall

Bethany qualified as a PNA in 2021 and led the implementation of the role into NHS Blood and Transplant, who have since been able to achieve the 1:20 PNA to nurse ratio laid out by NHS England. Bethany is now undertaking her PhD at Coventry University on the topic of the PNA role, focusing on how it can be sustained to continue driving meaningful, system-level improvements in a changing political healthcare landscape.
Bethany is passionate about building compassionate cultures and championing compassionate leadership to create an empowered and fulfilled nursing workforce. This chapter was important to Bethany as it covers not only compassionate cultures and leadership but also self-compassion. Nurses cannot go on looking after others without first looking after themselves. One of her favourite things about the PNA role is that it is about nurses, nursing nurses.

Laura Wilde

Dr Laura Wilde is a Research Psychologist specialising in digital health and psychosocial interventions for people with long-term health conditions. Her research focuses on co-producing inclusive, evidence-based resources that support well-being and self-management. As a Research Fellow at Coventry University, she contributed to the SUpervision, Support & Advocacy for Improvement in Nursing (SUSTAIN-ING) study, which explored the impact of Professional Nurse Advocates (PNAs) on patient outcomes and experiences through quality improvement initiatives. Working alongside nurses gave her a deep appreciation for the incredible work they do and the significance of the PNA role. Laura collaborated with Bethany Hall on the book chapters to emphasise the importance of well-being for both staff and patients.

Foreword

Since its introduction in 2021, the professional nurse advocate (PNA) role has added a vital new dimension to our nursing workforce. It represents a demonstrative and compassionate approach to supporting one another – creating space for reflection on our experiences in practice and fostering thoughtful improvements in how we meet the challenges of our work and care for our patients.

This book is the first to bring together a diverse range of voices, ideas, case examples that illustrate how the PNA role is being applied across different settings. It serves as a trusted companion with practical tools – a source of guidance, inspiration and reassurance that none of us face these challenges alone. Whether you are new to the role or have been practising as a PNA for some time, you will find something here that resonates, supports and strengthens your journey.

Across eight chapters, this book weaves together short case studies from practice with broader reflections on the origins and purpose of the PNA role. It explores the A-EQUIP model, nurse identity and belonging, and the leadership frameworks that enable PNAs and the nurses they work with to flourish. Central to these discussions is restorative clinical supervision – the heart of the PNA role. More recently, the focus on quality improvement has grown, and this is reflected in a dedicated chapter. The book concludes with insights into building communities of practice and cultivating compassion – essential elements in sustaining ourselves and our teams.

At a time when staff well-being and retention remain critical priorities, this book highlights how the PNA role helps us focus on what truly matters: listening, supporting and creating the conditions for reflection and growth. When we do these things well, we see tangible improvements – in how colleagues feel at work, in how they choose to stay, lead and care, and ultimately in the quality and safety of the care we deliver. PNAs play an integral role in sustaining the well-being of the nursing workforce and shaping a compassionate culture within health care.

I hope this book serves as a valuable resource for all involved in nursing education and practice. My sincere thanks go to everyone who has contributed to this work and to the wider PNA community. Your commitment, generosity and willingness to share your experiences continue to make an enduring difference.

Sophie Mayes
Lead PNA – Northampton General Hospital
Chair Systemwide PNA Forum
Vice Chair Midlands Professional Advocate Shared
Decision-Making Council

List of Abbreviations

ABC	Adaptive Behavioural Components
A-EQUIP	Advocating for Education and Quality Improvement
BME	Black and Minority Ethnic
CoPs	Communities of Practice
HEI	Health Education Institute
IEN	Internationally Educated Nurses
NHS	National Health Service
NMC	Nursing Midwifery Council
NQN	Newly Qualified Nurses
PMA	Professional Midwifery Advocate
PNA	Professional Nurse Advocate
QI	Quality Improvement
RCN	Royal College of Nursing
RCS	Restorative Clinical Supervision
RBCS	Resilience-Based Clinical Supervision

Keywords

collaboration
communities of practice
compassionate cultures
compassionate leadership
emotional labour
emotional intelligence
empathy
empowerment
evolving leadership theories
global nurse identity
nurse empowerment
professional nurse advocate
professional midwifery advocate
psychological safety
quality improvement
restorative clinical supervision
supervision
supervisors
supervisees
well-being

Acknowledgement for PNA Handbook

The editors would like to extend their huge gratitude and thanks to Heather Price, Associate Director of Nursing for Education and Research, and Amy Kelsey, senior sister (in critical care) and professional nurse advocate at University Hospitals Coventry and Warwickshire NHS Trust for the significant input to case studies within the Leadership Chapter by Jill Barr.

CHAPTER 1

Introducing PNA and PMA Developments

Emma Wadey[1] and Clare Capito[2]
[1]Queens Nursing Institute and American Academy of Nursing,
NHS Foundation Trust HERTFORDSHIRE England, London, UK
[2]NHS England, London, UK

INTRODUCTION

This chapter introduces the roles of the professional nurse advocate (PNA) and professional midwifery advocate (PMA), providing the context for their introduction into practice. It will reference relevant national policies, implementation guides, education standards and reporting mechanisms, supported by case studies that illustrate the application of these roles in practice. While the A-EQUIP (Advocating for Education and Quality Improvement) framework underpins both roles, the rationale for their development and initial implementation differs between nursing and midwifery. What remains consistent, however, is the shared recognition of the need to enable nursing and midwifery staff to pause, reflect and re-energise in response to the complex demands of their work.

The chapter will present key policies and evidence underpinning the roles and their functions, including the PNA and PMA A-EQUIP Implementation Guide and the RCN PNA Education Standards. It will also explore the development of the A-EQUIP model within the midwifery profession, the evolution of the PMA role in recent years and the growing collaboration between PMAs and their PNA counterparts.

THE CREATION AND DEVELOPMENT OF THE PROFESSIONAL MIDWIFERY ADVOCATE ROLE

In the United Kingdom, the midwifery profession has had a long history of supervision, which was initially set down in the Midwives Act of 1902. In that first iteration, the supervision of midwives was undertaken by inspectors who were not midwives, and their main role was to inspect the midwives' notes and equipment, as most births took place in women's homes. The role of inspection of midwives was one that did not provide support for midwives but was one that was more about the control and monitoring of a midwife's practice (Kirkham 1995).

Over the years, the model of supervision of midwives changed considerably and remained in statute until the end of March 2017. The supervision of midwives was largely focussed on a midwife's fitness to practise, whereby every midwife had to submit their intention to practise on an annual basis to their supervisor of midwives and in addition, if a midwife was involved in an incident, their clinical care could be investigated by a supervisor of midwives. If their midwifery practice was called into question, then the supervisor of midwives would recommend a remedial programme, which would be agreed upon by the Local Supervising Authority Midwifery Officer.

However, following the publication of the reports from the Parliamentary and Health Service Ombudsman (PHSO 2013) and the Department of Health (2016a,b) which both recommended that midwifery supervision and regulation should be separated, it was suggested that the Nursing Midwifery Council (NMC) should have direct control over the regulation of midwives and thus their fitness to practise.

When legislative changes took place on 31 March 2017, the statutory element of midwifery supervision, as well as the function of the Local Supervising Authorities (LSA) ceased to exist.

In 2016 and in preparation for the statutory and legislative changes, each of the four countries in the United Kingdom were tasked with establishing a time-limited taskforce to ensure processes of good clinical governance and support for midwifery practice.

In England, the taskforce consisted of stakeholders, which included women, midwives, academics, midwifery and nurse leaders, managers, commissioners and the Royal College of Midwives and Birthrights. A new model of midwifery supervision emerged from the consultation, known by its acronym as A-EQUIP and the PMA role was created to deploy the functions of the A-EQUIP model (NHS England 2018).

In April 2017, NHS England launched their new model of midwifery supervision, and its implementation was initially driven by the four Regional Maternity Teams and national oversight was from the Head of Maternity and her team in NHS England (NHS England 2018; Dunkley-Bent 2017).

TRAINING TO BECOME A PROFESSIONAL MIDWIFERY ADVOCATE

The PMA was a new role, and the principles of a curriculum had been developed by the task and finish group because the preparation was seen as essential to the success of delivering the A-EQUIP model (described fully in Chapter 4).

In November 2016, the first PMAs were trained in a pilot run by NHS England, which successfully trained 40 Supervisors of midwives to become PMAs, and by November 2018, there were 768 PMAs across the four regions of England in total.

Each region was responsible for procuring the PMA training courses and the London region co-designed the curriculum and assessment of the training programme with the four London university providers and Supervisors of Midwives. Each London Trust was allocated several training places to attend one of the four university providers and thus attend the same course and learn together as a team. The assessment consisted of each PMA team presenting an outline of the plan for how they would implement the PMA service in their organisation. This made the learning very practical, with a clear direction to their aims and objectives of the vision of their PMA service in their organisation.

Since 2020, NHS England has funded a total of 650 PMA training places, on average 150 places per year, to date. In April 2025, the National PMA Directory listed that there are 1592 qualified PMAs who work in NHS Trusts and non-NHS settings such as Higher Education Institutions (HEIs), pregnancy and abortion services and private maternity services.

Supporting Implementation of The PMA Role and Service

To support commissioners and providers in understanding the commissioning requirements of the A-EQUIP model, a specification was developed for the NHS Standard Contract in 2017/2018 and was mandated by NHS England for use by commissioners for all contracts for healthcare services other than primary care. In accordance with this contract, the provider must ensure that arrangements are in place for all midwives to receive the new national model of midwifery supervision. This specification remains in place and includes nurses as well as midwives to receive supervision as per the A-EQUIP model (NHS England 2021).

In order to support the development of the PMA role, each of the regions has set-up Regional PMA Support Networks and the case study below highlights how the North East and Yorkshire Regional PMA Support Network has achieved this:

Developing a Regional PMA Support Network

The North East and Yorkshire Regional PMA Support Network was established in 2020 and meets monthly on MS teams.

Sharing good practice and initiatives and challenges in a safe space among peers generates creativity, solutions and ideas, and this was the aim of the network.

Initially, within the network, we discussed the implementation of A-EQUIP across the region and shared:

- Good practice
- Challenges
- Involvement in the evaluation process
- Facilitated peer support

At the end of November 2023, it was agreed that we would seek feedback from the PMAs within the region around the benefit of the meeting and if it could be improved.

The PMAs in this group shared that they appreciated learning about the hard work, good work and challenges that their PMA peers were experiencing. They also fed back that this peer support was essential to the success of implementing and developing their PMA service.

It is apparent from the feedback and attendance that this is a valued forum for supporting PMAs within the region. The forum also gives the Regional Maternity Team opportunity to verbally express regularly the value that the support, compassion and leadership of PMAs provides and demonstrate the impact it has across the region.

Regional PMA Lead Roles in the Southeast

In 2023/2024 the Southeast Regional PMA co-leads wanted to meet with the PMAs in the region and discuss how the A-EQUIP model and PMA role were being implemented within their Trust. Therefore, they visited every Trust and found many excellent examples of practice reported by the PMA teams, including:

Supporting maternity staff well-being through 'Time for Tea', 'Hug in a Mug', crochet classes or during incident investigations quality improvement huddle boards and projects to support community midwives during homebirths; an induction of labour toolkit training and development opportunities such as trauma informed training practical elements of running the PMA service like 'PMA of the Day'.

As the A-EQUIP model is employer-led, there was variation noted among the Trusts in the Region in terms of its implementation, particularly around PMA leadership and organisational structure, processes and the availability of resources to undertake PMA activities. Challenges were also noted around securing protected time, staff engagement and understanding the A-EQUIP model. PMA teams continue to work to resolve the issues.

Following the visits, good practice principles were collated and the learning was shared at regional and national PMA forums. Further networking and collaboration opportunities have been created and restorative clinical supervision (RCS) sessions for PMA leads are now in place.

Charlotte Easton and Andrea Curling, Regional PMA Leads for the SE Region

In 2023/2024, the regional PMA leads in the Southeast of England visited all the PMA teams to provide in person, support to learn about their challenges and celebrate their successes as PMA teams. The Regional PMA leads developed a toolkit to assist these visits, and this toolkit has been further adapted for use by PMA teams across England whose maternity services are on the support programme and will be published in the forthcoming (2026) National Implementation Framework for the A-EQIUP model and PMA role.

Further Examples of Innovation and Improvements in Maternity Services Undertaken by PMAs

Over the last 8 years, PMAs across England have undertaken many initiatives in response to improvements in maternity services and below is an overview of several such initiatives.

PMA in Your Pocket: Simplifying Access to a PMA

Simplifying access to a PMA is essential. The dedicated email address was found to be a challenge for staff to access, i.e. lack of access to a computer to send an email.

A QR code can be scanned to complete a form to arrange a meeting with a PMA, and this QR code is found on a business card which fits in the back of a security pass or slips into a midwife's pocket – hence 'PMA in your pocket'.

Feedback has been good as it is simple to use and access a PMA. Due to the positive feedback, all student midwives and maternity support workers are provided with a card.

It's a simple system that anyone can set-up with great results!

Sarah McGrath, Lead PMA, Liverpool Women's Hospital

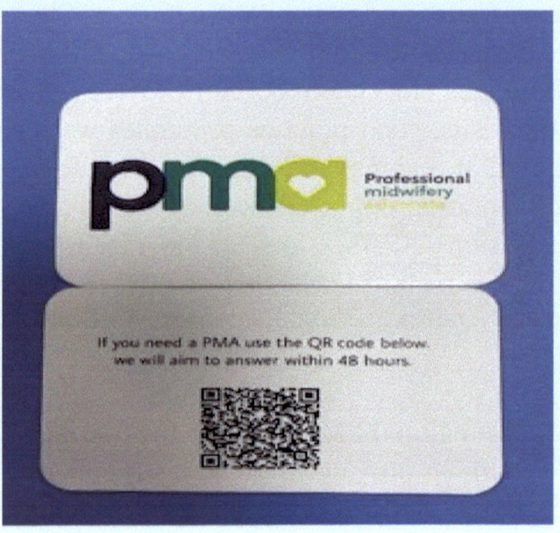

THE ACADEMIC PMA

The Academic PMA is an emerging role created initially by those lecturers who taught the PMA programme and by default have become PMAs.

Academic PMAs provide RCS to student midwives, which is very positively evaluated, and Kingston University has provided a case study of the 'Safe Spaces' that they have developed for their student midwives. In 2023, in recognition of this role, NHS England provided 50 PMA training places to midwifery lecturers to become academic PMAs in HEIs that do not provide PMA training but train midwifery students.

Implementing the PMA Role in a University to Support Student Midwives

At Kingston University, we are committed to maintaining safe spaces for all student midwives. The initial aim was to provide these spaces for students from marginalised groups, to discuss their experiences. Safe spaces can be described as environments where people, especially those from marginalised groups, can feel safe and respected and free from discrimination and these are led by the PMAs within the academic team.

The aim of 'safe spaces' is to empower students to speak up with our support to do this. Especially as there is awareness that these situations can affect physical and mental well-being if not addressed. Due to the positive feedback on the safe spaces, access has been rolled out to all students.

Students can discuss things that have affected them in clinical practice and often, it is only when they say it out loud that they begin to realise that they are describing things that can fit the descriptions for 'microaggressions', 'gaslighting' and 'othering'. However, when one person speaks up, it can give others the confidence to speak up too.

These safe spaces provide opportunities for student midwives to share their experiences in the learning environment which is led by a PMA who listens and encourages the students not to be silent bystanders, and that if they witness bad behaviour in practice, they should speak up, whether it was aimed at them or another student.

A further example from an academic PMA who recounts her experiences of teaching on the PMA course and listening to midwives and their positive accounts of the support they have received from a PMA is as follows:

As a lecturer and lead for a Professional Midwifery Advocacy (PMA) Course I have taught many midwives. The most striking thing for me facilitating this course is how much the midwives get personally from

(continued)

(*continued*)

attending the course. On the final teaching day, the students use representational art to help them discuss a challenging professional issue. The stories they bring are often traumatic and evoke a variety of emotions. The safe space of the cohort offers an opportunity for them to reflect in a way that they may not have had in the past and enables them to really appreciate the power of Restorative Clinical Supervision (RCS).

Over the course of this year, I recall 3 midwives who really stood out for me. These midwives had particularly difficult stories involving maternal care. One as a community midwife, was left with little support whilst caring for a woman with a complex obstetric history who had chosen to have a home birth 'out of guidance'. The second was part of an obstetric team faced with a situation of a woman and family who refused all intervention despite significant evolving picture of maternal decline. The third was more subtle but still challenging and involved her dismay of the changes in midwifery practice. The midwife found that the fear of litigation has negatively impacted her autonomy as a midwife and her ability to advocate for women. The midwife also commented that she believed that this was also affecting the declining morale of her midwifery colleagues.

Listening to these midwives and noting how helpful they found this exercise to be in allowing the space and time to talk was enough, but outside of this was the recognition from each of them of their own PMAs who had been there for them at these difficult times. Without exception they all spoke of how they were left 'burn out' and traumatised from events they had witness. All described their serious consideration to leave the profession and yet they are still practicing (one has been successful in a significant promotion). All are still midwives because of the support from their PMA teams who were there for them, offered time to talk through RCS, regularly checked in with them and signposted them to other support as required.

Capturing data about the importance of the role of the PMA is difficult but testimonies such as this must be heard; the significant power of this peer support cannot be understated.

An example of PMAs utilising themes from RCS sessions to develop an education tool for a birth phenomenon that is not well understood is as follows:

'Freebirthing – A Short Documentary': A QI Project Undertaken by PMAs

These PMAs were inspired to create this film in response to their work in understanding why midwives are leaving the profession and providing individual and group supervision sessions themed 'Challenges to providing birth outside of guidance.' Through these RCS sessions they identified themes such as confusion and lack of understanding about why women would choose to freebirth, with feelings of anger and fear about such choices, linked to fears about responsibility and liability. This demonstrated a need to find creative ways of educating both midwives and obstetricians about personalisation and choice in Maternity Services.

Freebirth or unassisted birth, as described by Birth Rights UK, means deciding to give birth without the attendance of a maternity healthcare professional such as a midwife. Personalisation and choice are a high priority on the NHS 3-year plan for maternity, however there are ongoing challenges in achieving these objectives. By using this phenomenon as a pure and extreme version of choice, we are encouraged to look at how we perceive choice and our biases about it.

The resulting film produced is being used as an education tool by many PMAs and lecturers throughout England and the feedback is extremely positive about a woman's choice which is not well understood.

In addition, this has led to further career opportunities for the PMAs to further study and teach about freebirth.

Josephine Ash and Jacq Crow, PMAs, Torbay and South Devon NHS Foundation Trust

THE CREATION AND DEVELOPMENT OF THE PROFESSIONAL NURSE ADVOCATE ROLE

In November 2020, the PNA programme was developed by the Head of Mental Health Nursing for England, Emma Wadey. In the early days of the Coronavirus Disease 2019 (COVID-19) outbreak, she recognised a significant knowledge–action gap in addressing nurses' well-being and their professional development. Feedback from registered nurses from the four fields of nursing practice and across healthcare settings, including hospital-based, community and mental health settings, highlighted their concerns about their invisibility and the lack of clinical supervision and opportunity to shape and influence patient care.

The research of the PMA role, programme and RCS, highlighted the following benefits: A reduction in sickness absence, increased staff satisfaction, improved patient experience, reduced turnover, improved team working relationships and increased recruitment of students, combined with an awareness of high rates of burnout, nurse suicide and poor retention. Given the PMA success and the need to support nurses, a business case was developed to implement the PNA programme. The PNA initiative was driven by nurses, acknowledging the importance of improving nurse well-being in increasing recruitment and retention and in improving patient care. The ambition was to build and sustain a health-based workplace culture in which nurses not only survive but thrive despite the complexities and demands of the role and potential exposure to vicarious trauma.

Launched by the former Chief Nursing Officer, Ruth May, in November 2020, the programme drew on the learning from the successful implementation of the PMA programme, which had been previously launched in 2017. In March 2021, the first PNA training programme commenced in Institutes of Higher Education across England. This was the start of a critical point of COVID-19 recovery – for patients, for services and for our workforce.

The PNA programme and the adoption of the A-EQUIP model of supervision (see Figure 1.1) have been the first of its kind for nursing, not just in England but across the world, as they equip staff who train as PNAs to listen and understand the challenges that fellow colleagues and teams are facing, and to provide and deliver quality improvement initiatives to improve patient care and staff well-being in response.

Professional nursing leadership and clinical supervision are essential in enabling nurses to continuously improve the care they provide to patients and their families, as well as to protect their own and their colleagues' health and well-being. The PNA role facilitates the elements of the A-EQUIP model of professional nursing leadership and clinical supervision.

TRAINING TO BECOME A PROFESSIONAL NURSE ADVOCATE

The PNA programme, taught at the master's degree level, is a postgraduate, professional leadership programme for registered nurses. It is designed to support psychological health and well-being, increase nurse retention and

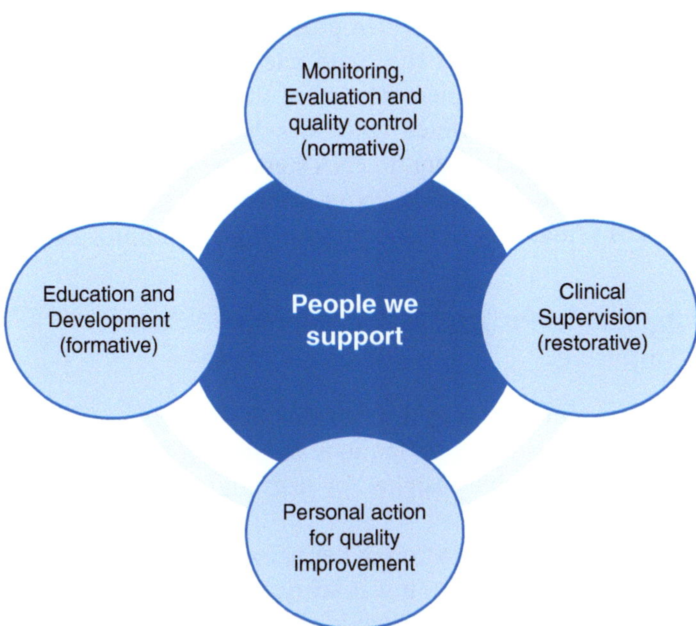

FIGURE 1.1   A-EQUIP model.

improve the quality of patient experiences. The programme is delivered across a growing number of HEIs across England.

On completion of the programme, nurses facilitate RCS, offer career coaching and lead quality improvement projects. Research has reported RCS addresses the emotional needs of staff, by reducing stress and burnout in staff, while career coaching offers the opportunity to discuss and plan career development and professional opportunities key to successful retention.

Supporting Implementation of The PNA Role and Service

Between 2021 and 2024, over 11,000 PNA training places were funded for nurses working across England and in the military, in all areas of clinical practice including hospital, community, primary care and criminal justice settings. Since data collection began in April 2022, the PNAs have delivered over 48,000 sessions of RCS to nursing colleagues, facilitated over 30,000 career conversations with nurses in practice and have led over 2200 quality improvement programmes to improve patient care each month. A further 1600 PNA training places have been funded by NHS England in 2025–2026, demonstrating the ongoing support of the PNA role.

Since the Launch of the PNA Programme in 2021, PMAs Have Worked Collaboratively with their PNAs Colleagues.

In the first few cohorts of the PNA programme, PMAs were utilised to provide support to student PNAs and some acted as their supervisors. This was pivotal to the successful implementation of the programme and cemented a collaborative partnership which continues in practice. Many PMAs have offered RCS training and support to PNA students. More recently, there was a push to increase the number of PNAs in neonatal services, and this is an example of PMAs and PNAs collaborating on a quality improvement initiative.

My Baby Labels Project: A Collaboration Between PMAs and PNAs

This case study demonstrates the role of both the PMA and PNA working collaboratively – listening to families to make a quality improvement as they provide valuable insights for learning and the development of maternity services.

Talking about the separation of her baby at birth one mother wrote, 'I felt disconnected from her ... it was scary, and I had thoughts of her not really being mine and I was just looking after someone else's baby ... surely this wasn't normal?' Another described looking across the NNU wondering which baby was hers as she saw nothing familiar in her baby, leading to delayed bonding.

During a NNU development day, which was facilitated by a PMA, these stories, were read out to the team. The reflection led to a deeper more considered discussion about the possibility of creating bespoke baby name labels for such families and a project called **'My Baby Labels'** was launched. **The project utilised Quality Improvement methodology and was led by a** newly qualified PNA from the neonatal team who was inspired to use his advocacy skills and was supported by PMAs through this improvement initiative.

My Baby Labels is a project where parents choose the labels prior to the birth of their baby; they choose the colour, write something in their own words on the label, and the label is attached to their baby immediately after birth and remains on the baby for the whole time that the parents are separated from their babies.

Prior to the launch of 'My Baby Labels' project, families were asked for their comments of the proposed project and reported that:

> *I wish we had this when my little girl was born, I still thought she wasn't mine for hours after we were together again.*

Sandra Pygott, Lead PMA & Dave Speck PNA, ULTH

THE PNA ROLE IN PRACTICE

The ambition at the launch of the PNA programme was to ensure every nurse in practice would have access to a PNA so that they could benefit from RCS, access career conversations and engage in quality improvement. To support the rollout, regional PNA leads were recruited, who facilitated the training places and supported organisations in identifying a senior nurse leader to champion the rollout of PNA within the organisation and ensure that all NHS settings had trained PNAs in practice.

The expectations for NHS regions, organisations, PNAs and nurses were set out in the co-produced publication 'Professional Nurse Advocate A-Equip Model: A model of clinical supervision for Nurses', published in 2021 by NHS England.

Training places, and the delivery of RCS, career conversations and quality improvements were reported via workforce returns with monthly oversight and monitoring to track progress of implementation. Research and evaluations were commissioned to measure impact, and monthly national webinars took place to share good practice across England.

Of note is that each organisation was supported in shaping their PNA offer to meet the needs of their specific area, ensuring an approach which was led and directly influenced by nurses. Examples in practice include PNA Duty service, as an initial response to supporting the workforce, and offering group and individual RCS, drop-in sessions, after-incident support, preceptorship sessions and partnership working with quality improvement leads.

Case Study: PNA in Action Managing Distress

I received a referral for a PNA session from a Team Leader about one of her Band 5 staff members. The staff member had submitted a resignation letter which had come out of the blue, and she was concerned. I arranged a virtual meeting with the staff member, who was currently on sick leave. I explained that although the referral came from the Team Leader, our conversation would be confidential.

The staff member was visibly distressed. They were dealing with personal issues that were impacting their mental health and affecting their ability to function at work. At that point, they felt resignation was the only way forward.

Through the application of the A-EQUIP model, I was able to provide a restorative space where the staff member could reflect on their situation, explore alternative options and consider pathways to support. We explored other options besides resignation and looked at ways they could access support for their mental health.

I followed up after the session. The staff member withdrew their resignation, accessed the support they needed and began to resolve the personal issues they were facing. They are now in a leadership role and still working within the Trust.

This experience reminded me of the importance of the PNA role – being able to offer a restorative space, listen without judgement and support staff to find a way forward when things feel overwhelming.

IMPACT OF PNA

Benefits included providing a framework for the consistent delivery of effective and psychological safe clinical supervision, delivering professional development at Level 7 (master's level), with recognised national qualification in leadership and advocacy and equipping nurses to ensure continuous quality improvement in practice to improve patient experience and outcomes.

The positive impact of the programme for those undertaking the course was immediate; most of those early pioneers had been considering leaving the profession but were now committed to stay and work collectively to improve the work experience of nursing and wider healthcare colleagues. Specifically, it was reported that the facilitation of RCS in healthcare settings was transformative.

The development of PNAs in practice settings helps nurses feel valued and empowered. The programme has ensured access to RCS and opened opportunities for nurses to engage in further study and development. Implementation requires time for PNAs to be trained, and time in practice for them to conduct the role within the clinical setting. The 'PNA movement', has transformed nursing practice, highlighting the importance of RCS for staff well-being and clinical effectiveness and the contribution of nurses in the recovery of services post-COVID-19. The following case study is a good illustration.

Case Study: Restorative Support for Nurse Involved in Patient Deterioration Incident

A Band 5 nurse was involved in a significant incident where a deteriorating patient suffered harm. There were delays in escalation due to gaps in practice, and although this was a system-level issue, the experience left the nurse deeply distressed. She reported feeling overwhelmed, guilty and fearful about the ongoing investigation. More than anything, she feared judgement from her team and began to question her clinical competence and future in the profession.

A referral was made to a Professional Nurse Advocate (PNA) who was based outside of the nurse's Division, which immediately helped create a safe, neutral space for reflection and support. Initially, only one restorative clinical supervision (RCS) session was arranged. However, the session proved so helpful that the nurse requested two additional sessions.

In the first session, she became emotional and said it was the first time she felt she could speak honestly. She had been internalising a sense of failure and feeling isolated. The PNA helped her reflect on the wider context of the incident, validate her emotional response, and explore how she could access further support.

In the subsequent sessions, they worked together to rebuild her confidence, understand her reactions and reframe her professional identity. The PNA also signposted her to well-being services and helped identify local allies for peer support.

The nurse later expressed how grateful she was for the time and space to talk and reflect. She shared that the support helped her to feel more confident and prepared to re-engage with her role.

This case illustrates the powerful role PNAs play in supporting staff well-being following patient safety incidents, especially when offered in a psychologically safe and neutral environment.

Binsy Mathew
Practice Development Lead Nurse (Cross Site)
Lewisham and Greenwich NHS Trust

The following points summarise the key programme deliverables to date:

- Over 11,000 training places have been commissioned by NHS England from March 2021 to March 2024.
- 2120 psychological booster sessions have been offered to all qualified PNAs between November 2021 and March 2024.

- Eleven national webinars have taken place between March 2021 and December 2023, sharing good practice and learning, reaching 4430 attendees.
- Commissioning of further continued professional development opportunities, including motivational interviewing, compassionate leadership and mindfulness.
- PNA evaluation, independent PNA research and PNA PhD opportunity starting in early 2024.
- Updated National PNA Guidance (October 2023).
- Royal College of Nursing PNA Standards.
- NHS contract.
- E-Learning modules on the role of PNA and the A-EQUIP model as well as the PMA role.
- PNA webpages and PNA Future NHS Platform.

Provider Workforce Returns (PWR) data is submitted monthly to NHS England, which indicates how many RCS sessions and career conversations have been facilitated by PNAs, and how many quality improvement projects/programmes are currently underway led and supported by PNAs, as well as the number of PNAs in post. Since September 2023, PMAs have also been collecting their activity data via PWR, utilising the same metrics.

Key Programme Outcomes

- 44,826 restorative clinical sessions have been conducted by PNAs between April 2022 and November 2023.
- 27,950 career conversations have been delivered by PNAs between September 2022 and November 2023.
- 2087 quality improvement projects/programmes are currently underway in November 2023, supported by PNAs.
- PNAs support nurses with their own mental health and well-being as well as the mental health and well-being of their healthcare colleagues.

A national report, which included a rapid review of published evidence available at the time demonstrated that the PNA programme meets the criteria for effective clinical supervision and that RCS has well-being benefits, including a reduction in reported stress and burnout and improvements in compassion satisfaction (Lees-Deutsch et al., 2023).

SUMMARY

The roles of PMA and PNA have been pivotal in transforming professional practice across England. The recognition of the importance of RCS in practice to support the well-being of health staff and improve recruitment and retention has ensured that nurses and midwives have the tools and resources to support, shape and influence care. The success of both programmes has been sustained through collaborative working between professions and the continued positive impact the roles are having on staff.

> ### Case Study: Using the A-EQUIP Model
>
> In a recent one-on-one RCS session, using the A-EQUIP framework, I met a junior nursing colleague who is currently undertaking academic studies. She initiated the session to discuss her interest in joining the nursing bank for additional night shifts – a decision she hoped to move forward with by gaining my support and sign-off.
>
> We began by revisiting our safe space agreement, reinforcing confidentiality, respect and emotional safety. She was already familiar with this set-up, and the session was held in a pre-booked room with minimal interruptions. What was new, however, was the introduction of a mindfulness exercise. I guided her through a brief breathing exercise, followed by a mental body scan in a relaxed seated position. This gentle centring helped her settle into the reflective process that followed.
>
> To explore her emotional state, we used a 'blob tree' image – a playful, yet profound tool. She selected the 'blob' clinging by its fingertips to a branch, an indicator of emotional strain. When prompted, she shared how the ongoing impact of the pandemic had left her family in financial difficulty. Her partner had been furloughed for a long period, with two small children and the shame of borrowing money from family members, it seemed the burden had fallen disproportionately on her shoulders. The need to take on bank shifts came not from professional ambition, but from a profound sense of responsibility to her family.
>
> Our conversation began to shift from the logistics of temporary bank work to the emotional undercurrents driving her decision. Despite academic excellence – her results consistently exceeding 80% – she had recently taken two episodes of sick leave. This prompted a deeper reflection on her well-being. We explored the possible consequences of 'falling from the tree', and how this imagery paralleled her internal state.

Using the 'responsibility pie' tool, we visualised how much of the current pressure was truly hers to carry. She acknowledged that no more than 50% of the burden was hers, and that her self-imposed expectations were contributing to her emotional exhaustion. We discussed the overlapping roles she held – mother, wife, student, and daughter – and how often self-care slipped from view when meeting everyone else's needs.

By the end of the session, the supervisee had shifted from a singular goal of getting a sign-off, to a more nuanced and compassionate plan of action. She decided to revisit the financial situation with her partner and together evaluate whether night shifts were truly necessary. She expressed that this was the first time she had voiced these thoughts out loud, and that previously, all her decision-making had remained internal.

Her feedback was poignant – she felt clearer and lighter, describing the space as somewhere she could finally 'breathe'. She realised that presenting a pre-decided plan to her partner may have ignored the opportunity for collaboration and mutual understanding. Importantly, I too reflected on my own responsibilities. Had I simply signed off the request, it could have been perceived as permission. This session reaffirmed the importance of engaging with the person – not just the professional.

One tangible takeaway for me: Always bring tissues. Emotions surfaced unexpectedly, and Whilst I had to briefly leave to retrieve some, I'd prefer to remain present in moments of vulnerability. Emotionally charged restorative supervision demands preparedness, not just procedural readiness.

This session embodied the NMC Code themes – particularly *Prioritise People*. We didn't just address her professional situation but honoured her emotional reality. In doing so, we practised compassion, broke down assumptions and strengthened trust.

REFERENCES

Department of Health (2016a). Proposals for changing the system of midwifery supervision in the UK. London, DH.

Department of Health (2016b). National Maternity Review. Better Births. Improving outcomes of maternity services in England. A five year forward review for maternity care. (Chair: Cumberlege, J.), London, DH. http://www.england.nhs.uk/wp-content/uploads/2016/02/national-maternity-review-report.pdf (accessed 22 December 2025).

Dunkley-Bent, J. (2017). A-EQUIP: the new model of midwifery supervision. *British Journal of Midwifery* 25: 5.

Kirkham, M. (1995). The history of midwifery supervision. *Super-Vision: Consensus Conference Proceedings.* Ed. Association of Radical Midwives.

Lees-Deutsch, L., Adegboye Rodrigues Amorim, A., Bayes, N. et al. (2023). *National Evaluation Report of the Professional Nurse Advocate Programme in England.* Coventry University https://doi.org/10.18552/RIHW/2023/0001.

NHS England (2018) A-EQUIP advocating for education and quality improvement, England's model of midwifery supervision—'one year on'. https://www.england.nhs.uk/wp-content/uploads/2018/09/aequip-one-year-on-report.pdf (accessed 18 March 2025).

NHS England (2021). *Professional Nurse Advocate A-Equip Model: A Model of Clinical Supervision for Nurses.* London: NHS England.

Parliamentary Health Service Ombudsman (2013). *Midwifery Supervision: Recommendations for Change.* London: The Stationary Office https://www.ombudsman.org.uk/sites/default/files/Midwifery%20supervision%20and%20regulation_%20recommendations%20for%20change.pdf.

CHAPTER 2

Nurse Identity, Global Belonging and the Professional Nurse Advocate Role

Analisa Smythe

The Royal Wolverhampton NHS Trust, Faculty of Research and Clinical Education Cavell Close, UK
Research and Development, Birmingham and Solihull Mental Health Foundation Trust, Birmingham, UK
Staffordshire University, School of Health, Education, Policing and Sciences, UK
Nottingham Trent University, School of Health Sciences, UK

Learning Points

1. Nurses all over the world view themselves as a unified global health community, with a shared sense of professional identity and common values and ideals.

2. Organisations can foster nurse identity and belonging through positive communication, supportive teams and inclusive leadership.

3. The PNA is in a unique position to promote nurse identity and belonging.

4. Nurses at all levels need to feel that they belong.

CONCEPTS OF GLOBAL NURSE IDENTITY

Nursing differs significantly across countries due to variations in cultural, social, healthcare and economic systems (International Nurses Council, ICN 2020). Despite these differences, many nurses all over the world view themselves as a unified global health community, with a shared sense of professional identity, common values and ideals centred on patient care (Van der Cingel and Brouwer 2021). Professional identity refers to an individual's self-concept as a professional nurse and includes beliefs, behaviours and values, related to honesty, compassion, respect and integrity. Nurses develop professional identity through a complex socialisation process that includes education, clinical experiences, interactions with colleagues' patients and their families, as well as exposure to professional values (Hill 2023; Hinkley et al. 2023). In most high- to middle-income countries, nurse education will involve a bachelor's degree, although in some countries, including Asia, Africa and South America, nurse education still includes several diploma or certificate programmes. A longitudinal study by Ho (2025) suggested that nurses gradually internalise professional values and transition from one identity to another over time, with students entering nurse education with existing personal identities, being socialised into the profession, and becoming fully integrated into the role, e.g. 'thinking and acting' like a nurse. Benner's novice to expert theory also focuses on the development of skills and knowledge, highlighting the differences between applied and theoretical knowledge (Benner 1984). Once newly qualified nurses (NQNs) understand their roles and develop expertise, they can learn the essential values, behaviours and skills required in the nursing profession. Mastery of the role demonstrates NQNs commitment to both their professional proficiencies, the Code and the organisation, and is also associated with increased motivation as individuals feel more competent in their role (Baharum et al. 2023; Deci and Ryan 1985).

When personal values and beliefs align, conscious motivation is strengthened. The values and beliefs about nursing which motivate nurses to enter the profession and beliefs about nursing are crucial in guiding professional behaviour (Poorchangizi et al. 2017). These values form the ethical foundation of nursing practice, influencing decision-making, communication and care delivery. When organisational culture and values are not aligned with personal ideals, individuals may feel they cannot practice in line with their personal values and beliefs, so they may choose to leave the profession (Ho et al. 2021). A well-established professional identity can promote open communication and effective decision-making, protecting nurses from moral injury and ensuring the confidence to challenge others when encountering conflict. Ensuring nurses develop a strong sense of professional identity early in their careers can mitigate against transition shock and help reduce stress and prevent burnout (Hinkley et al. 2023; Sabancıogullari and Dogan 2015).

Developing a strong professional identity can be challenging, as although many nurses perceive themselves to be relatively autonomous leaders, the social significance of the profession and the image of nurses remains ambiguous and potentially globally devalued (Woldasemayat et al. 2022). In South Asia and Africa, nurses may face cultural perceptions that mean nursing is less socially valued compared to other healthcare professions (Ndirangu et al. 2021). In other countries, such as Japan, nursing is closely aligned with cultural expectations of familiar care and support (Hirata and Harvath 2016). Cultural expectations of patient care and approaches to patient autonomy also differ in some Eastern countries (Jenkins and Smythe 2024). Even in Western countries where nursing is viewed as a respected profession, negative public perceptions persist, with nursing often viewed as an acquiescent 'feminine' gendered profession (Van der Cingel and Brouwer 2021).

More recently, nurses have been idealised as self-sacrificing 'heroes', leading to unrealistic expectations and a lack of support for nurses' health and well-being (Mohammed et al. 2018). In a discussion paper exploring nursing identity and misrepresentation of nursing in the media, Garcia and Qureshi (2024) suggest that nurse identity is given to nurses, rather than developed from within the profession, and that personal identity is diminished when there is conflict between personal insiders' experience (of being a nurse) and outsiders (public). This may be exacerbated when family members lack respect for the profession, often linked to poor public perceptions (López-Verdugo et al. 2021). Addressing the public perception of nursing is therefore critical, as positive personal identity can attract new nurses to the profession and encourage them to stay in nursing. In contrast, negative public perceptions may deter individuals from joining an already depleted workforce.

A SENSE OF BELONGING IN NURSING

West et al. (2020) defined belonging as 'the need to be connected to, cared for, and caring of others around them at work, and to feel valued, respected and supported' (p. 6). The core components of belonging include the perception of being part of a team (Clarke et al. 2020), a connection to the community and access to socio-emotional support (Reinhardt et al. 2020). Other features of belonging include a sense of autonomy and the need to feel trusted, valued and accepted (Patel et al. 2024). A supportive environment is characterised by effective teams with shared leadership and by relationships which promote respect, honesty, open communication and collaboration (Patel et al. 2024; West et al. 2020).

Belonging is essential for all social beings, but the concept becomes especially important in high-stress environments like health care. Belonging is associated with well-being, confidence, job satisfaction and morale (Hill 2024). Additionally, a sense of belonging positively relates to commitment to professional development (Allen et al. 2021). A strong sense of belonging improves relationships, fosters positive social skills and creates a sense of solidarity that translates to professional growth, enhanced performance at work and retention. Hill (2024) suggests that a sense of belonging is associated with cohesive teams, which can offer opportunities to reflect on difficult experiences at work and lead to improvements in psychological and social well-being (Hill 2024). Conversely, in teams which exhibit fewer teamwork behaviours, nurses experience increased loneliness, isolation and disconnection, associated with workplace conflicts, reduced confidence, stress and burnout (Frangieh et al. 2024; Patel et al. 2024). High-volume workloads, cultural barriers, transition periods and workplace dynamics such as bullying, incivility, conflict, exclusion or a lack of support can all erode a sense of belonging (West et al. 2020). Teamwork is essential to protecting patients, and research has found that poor teamwork increases the risk of patient complications and death (Mazzocco et al. 2009).

THE GLOBAL WORKFORCE

The COVID-19 pandemic highlighted the global shortage of qualified nurses, which is a significant challenge for healthcare systems worldwide, negatively impacting patient outcomes (Health and Social Care Select Committee 2022), as well as nurses themselves, with shortages leading to higher workloads, associated with stress and burnout (Collard et al. 2020; Buchan and Catton 2023). This shortage, estimated at 29 million nurses worldwide (Boniol et al. 2022), is related to a range of factors, including increases in the ageing population, demand for healthcare services, an ageing workforce, poor workforce planning and increased international recruitment, which has further exacerbated nursing shortages (Drennan and Ross 2019). Nurse retention is also showing signs of worsening (Collard et al. 2020) and is acknowledged as a worldwide concern (NHS Digital 2018). The NHS Long-Term Plan (2023) sets out plans for the expansion of the domestic workforce, culture change to improve retention and the creation of new roles, so that staff can spend more time with patients. The plan aims to ensure fewer staff leave over the next 15 years by improving workplace culture, leadership, well-being and flexible working, including pension reforms and childcare support. Research has shown that improving staffing levels and increasing nurse autonomy and involvement in decision-making have led to nursing becoming a more attractive profession in the United States (Health Foundation 2019). The recent policy document, the 10 Year Health Plan for England: fit for the future, sets out plans to ensure NHS staff will be better treated, more motivated, have better training and more scope to develop their careers in the future (Department of Social Care 2025).

Internationally Educated Nurses

Nursing shortages are disproportionately low in low- and middle-income countries; however, low numbers of graduate nurses and existing shortages have led many high-income countries, such as the United Kingdom and the United States, to rely on international nursing mobility (Lanada and Culligan 2024). Nurses tend to migrate to richer Western countries motivated by better pay, working conditions and career opportunities (Peters et al. 2020). In addition to nurses choosing to move for economic reasons, many nurses experience involuntary migration as refugees, displaced by conflict. In 2022, 108.4 million people worldwide were displaced because of violence, conflict and persecution, and with ongoing unrest in Ukraine and Palestine, these numbers continue to grow (The UN Refugee Agency 2023). Chang Chiu et al. (2024) suggest many of these are highly qualified professionals, although there is limited data on nurse displacement in conflict zones.

While labour shortages should mean that internationally educated nurses (IENs) have considerable leverage and rights to demand fair and good working conditions and access to professional development opportunities (Laing and Smythe 2024), the literature suggests that international status impacts negatively on career advancement and development opportunities (Lanada and Culligan 2024). IENs often experience cultural displacement; it can be challenging to integrate into new healthcare environments, as even if the foreign language is similar, differences in organisational structures, nursing practice, roles and autonomy mean that many feel like 'outsiders' in their host country (Pressley et al. 2022; Zizzo and Xu 2009).

The Nursing Workforce in the United Kingdom

The NHS depends on its workforce to deliver safe and effective care; however, nearly 10% of the current nursing workforce are considering leaving the profession (Health Education England 2020). The NHS Long-Term Workforce Plan aims to address critical nursing shortages, support retention and meet the growing needs of the UK population (NHS England 2023a, b, c; 2025, Fit for the future). The plan focuses on increasing staff numbers and retaining existing talent, reducing dependency on international recruitment, expanding education pathways, promoting apprenticeships and shorter training programmes, improving staff retention and well-being and modernising roles and expanding scopes of practice, with enhanced roles for nurses and allied health professionals (AHPs) (NHS England 2023a, b, c). The NHS plan also includes specific strategies for NQN retention such as mentorship, career development and better working conditions (NHS England 2023a, b, c).

In 2018, there were more nurses exiting the profession than joining the UK workforce (NHS Digital 2018), with NQNs leaving the profession at a higher rate than in any other year of experience. However, retention rates are changing; in 2025, staff leaving the NHS, including nurses, was among the lowest in over a decade (NHS England 2025). These retention improvements are attributed, in part, to the People Promise staff retention programme (NHS England 2021), which includes interventions like flexible working, improved opportunities for learning and well-being initiatives. Notwithstanding, a fifth of the nursing and midwifery profession are leaving within 10 years of joining the register (Kings Fund 2024). NQNs, minoritised groups and nurses nearing retirement are the groups most likely to leave. The transition from nursing student to qualified nurse can be a particularly challenging time; some NQNs report feeling unprepared and ill-equipped for the role. NQNs can face unrealistic expectations from senior staff, may struggle with role clarity and feel that they do not receive adequate support (Smythe and Carter 2022). These factors combined can lead to stress, contributing to job dissatisfaction and intention to leave the profession. Much of the existing research into the transition experiences of NQNs has been conducted internationally (Hawkins et al. 2018), pre-COVID-19. Nevertheless, low confidence, in combination with an unsupportive working environment, has been identified as the main factor influencing NQNs' decisions to leave nursing (Lee and De Gagne 2022).

The NHS workforce is becoming increasingly more diverse, with Black and minority ethnic (BME) nurses, midwives and health visitors making up almost a third (29.2%) of the workforce (NHS England 2023a, b, c).

The number of BME board members across all NHS trusts has increased to 13.2% in 2022. Pre-pandemic data shows attrition among overseas-qualified staff varies by country of origin and staff role; however, the reasons for this are uncertain (Kelly et al. 2002). Even less is known about attrition among staff from ethnic minority groups who have qualified in the United Kingdom. Notwithstanding, staff from minoritised groups are more likely to experience lower pay and poorer career progression (Buchan et al. 2019). In a recent survey of NHS leaders from ethnic minority groups, over half reported discrimination and exclusion (BME Leadership Network, 2022).

STRATEGIES TO SUPPORT NURSE IDENTITY AND BELONGING

Organisations can foster nurse identity and belonging through positive communication, supportive teams and inclusive leadership, ensuring all staff feel respected, regardless of background or experience (West et al. 2020). A range of specific interventions have also been found to improve nurse identity and belonging. These include interventions suitable for the wider nursing workforce, such as peer support programmes, clinical supervision, mentorship and wellness activities, and more specific interventions for IENs and NQNs, such as diversity and communication skills training and preceptorship.

Resources

National preceptorship framework for nursing `https://www.england.nhs.uk/long-read/national-preceptorship-framework-for-nursing/`

Supervision guidance for primary care network multidisciplinary teams

`https://www.england.nhs.uk/long-read/supervision-guidance-for-primary-care-network-multidisciplinary-teams/`

Supported self-management: peer support guide. `https://www.england.nhs.uk/long-read/peer-support`

Support for Internationally Educated Nurses

Despite the large numbers of international nurses working in countries such as the United States and England, there has been limited attention to supporting acculturation and the long-term retention of this important component of the nursing workforce (Chang Chiu et al. 2024). The responsibility for successful integration should not solely lie with the IENs but with recruiting organisations and wider teams, e.g. colleagues and managers. Systematic reviews have highlighted the need for organisations to include training to raise awareness of the challenges faced by IENs related to racism, marginalisation, bullying, discrimination and limited career opportunities, with many IENs prevented from utilising existing knowledge and expertise (Bond et al. 2020; Lanada and Culligan 2024). Hostile interactions with patients and colleagues have been shown to undermine belonging and identity, negatively impacting IENs' overall well-being at work (Chang Chiu et al. 2024; Dahl et al. 2022).

Successful cultural integration requires input from both IENs and nurses from the host country (Roth et al. 2021). Several papers on this topic have indicated that the transition process involves two-way learning and opportunities for cultural integration (Pung and Goh 2017; Shen et al. 2012; Davda et al. 2018; Cummins 2009). Therefore, successful integration requires all staff to be prepared, engaged, adequately informed and aware of the challenges that negatively impact IENs' practice. The NHS equality, diversity and inclusion improvement plan (2023a, b, c) aims to improve equality, diversity and inclusion and to enhance the sense of belonging for NHS staff. This includes plans for more inclusive recruitment and career progression. There has been an increase in representation of BME nurses, midwives and health visitors at board level, including executive board roles; however, the staff remain proportionally under-represented in senior positions, which is why the Long-Term Plan asked every NHS trust to set targets for senior BME representation reflective of their overall workforce (NHS England 2023a, b, c).

The literature suggests communication plays a key role in the acculturation and integration of IENs. This may reflect the complexity and nuanced nature of effective communication. Linguistic challenges can negatively impact IENs' sense of belonging, leading to interpersonal conflict and feelings of exclusion, disempowerment and isolation (Chang Chiu et al. 2024). Language and communication barriers were the most frequently cited concern of employers, regulatory bodies and nurses themselves (Pung and Goh 2017) although the language capabilities of IENs may receive undue scrutiny and errors attributed uncritically to language difficulties (Bond et al. 2020). A recent study by Kamau et al. (2023) suggested that adapting to the linguistic limitations of IENs can lead to an improved sense of nurse belonging.

Several studies included in a review by Dahl et al. (2022) exploring migration motives and integration commented on the cultural environment and the need to acquire soft skills, associated with a holistic model of care rather than a curative one. Indeed, expectations regarding critical thinking, independent decision-making and advocating are key aspects of nursing care in most contexts, which may add further complexity (Bond et al. 2020). Hence, the requirement for support interventions that promote an empathetic style of communication, confidence, autonomy and self-efficacy (Dahl et al. 2022; Laing and Smythe 2024). Examples may include considering the education and any culture-specific expectations of IENs, and adapting teaching styles and input accordingly, as well as encouraging transcultural exchange to share good practice and using role play focusing on clinical scenarios; however, there is a lack of research exploring support interventions for IENs (Laing and Smythe 2024).

The literature highlights the need for both informal and formal structured support for IENs. Informal support and connections with peers can make a positive and significant difference in personal confidence and acculturation. Peer support can increase emotional resilience, workplace integration and professional development (Bond et al. 2020). The findings of the review by Lanada and Culligan (2024) suggest that peer support and mentorship should be considered a critical element within support programmes, which should be offered for the first year of working in the host country.

Newly Qualified Nurses

Inclusive work environments that foster a culture where NQNs feel valued, respected and included are critical during the transition phase from student to NQN (Smythe and Carter 2022). NQNs frequently experience transition shock, associated with stress burnout, and feelings of inadequacy and self-doubt (John 2019). Supporting NQNs in building their professional identity and sense of belonging is essential for developing professional confidence and clinical effectiveness (Aldosari et al. 2020). Approval from colleagues and peers appears to be a major cause of stress, as most NQNs have a desire to become acknowledged and accepted within their workplace (Smythe and Carter 2022; Craig and Machin 2020). Research suggests that a lack of belonging and a sense of 'not fitting in' leads to a reduction in confidence levels (Austin and Halpin 2021). Research suggests that creating a culture of belonging for NQNs through supportive relationships with preceptors, mentors and peers is essential for a successful transition (Craig and Machin 2020).

Specific interventions to facilitate nurse identity and belonging include structured orientation and preceptorship programmes, which can help introduce NQNs to workplace culture and policies, create a supportive culture and provide emotional support (Mansour and Mattukoyya 2019). Professional development and opportunities for reflection can also be effective as they enhance skills, build confidence and clarify clinical expectations (Smythe and Carter 2022). Other strategies to support nurse identity and belonging include providing opportunities and creating spaces where belonging and cohesion can occur (Allen et al. 2021). These include team-building activities, social events, check-ins and huddles, with the whole team having protected time to have lunch or coffee breaks together (West et al. 2020). However, the effectiveness of interventions relies on their quality and delivery. Interventions that are not delivered as intended can heighten loneliness and isolation (Bodey 2024). Supporting student nurses' sense of belonging is also critical for improving retention, learning by applying knowledge and well-being. Nursing identity through clinical placements can be enhanced by integrating opportunities that increase belongingness (Squire et al. 2024). Specific strategies include mentorships and peer support schemes, buddy systems or student communities (e.g. ethnic minority nursing societies).

Strategies to Support Nurse Identity and Belonging

1. Team-building activities, e.g. coffee mornings
2. Social get-togethers, e.g. huddles or shared lunches
3. Protected lunch and coffee breaks
4. Creating spaces where social activities can take place
5. Opportunities for reflection, e.g. clinical supervision

THE PROFESSIONAL NURSE ADVOCATE ROLE

The PNA role, introduced in the United Kingdom following the COVID-19 pandemic and deploying the A-EQUIP model, is designed to empower nurses, promote education and development, build personal and professional resilience using a restorative approach, enhance the quality of patient care and support preparedness for appraisal and revalidation (Ariss et al. 2017). The PNA is in a unique position to promote nurse identity and belonging.

Professional Identity and Empowerment

The PNA role can reinforce professional identity and' belonging by empowering and supporting nurses to develop self-confidence and a culture of autonomy, where nurses at all levels feel valued and are empowered to contribute to change, quality improvement and innovation (Lees-Deutsch et al. 2023, 2025; Smythe et al. 2023). Enablement and empowerment are associated with increased levels of self-efficacy and positive work feelings, including improved job satisfaction, organisational commitment and staff morale (Lees-Deutsch et al. 2023).

Nurse Well-being

Informal evaluations of the PNA role suggest nurses who receive restorative clinical supervision (RCS) benefit emotionally and are more equipped to cope with challenges within the clinical area (Griffiths 2022; Wade 2023). A study by Smythe et al. (2023) exploring the impacts of the PNA role reported that RCS was perceived as helping to facilitate a solution-focused approach to problem-solving and develop an individual's reflective understanding of a situation.

Impact on PNA Supervisor

There are also accounts of the impact on PNA supervisors, which suggest that the PNA role has the potential to revive nursing careers and create additional opportunities to support colleagues (Pearce 2023; Hogan 2023). The study by Smythe et al. (2023) reported that practising PNAs experience a wide range of impacts, including an increased sense of empowerment, commitment to the role, role fulfilment and personal accomplishment. The National Evaluation by Lees-Deutsch et al. (2023) also recognised that the PNA programme creates opportunities for nurses to engage in further study and development, which may develop transferable leadership and interpersonal skills.

IMPLICATIONS FOR HEALTH AND POLICY

Policies at all levels are required to promote an inclusive and supportive workplace culture that values equity, good working conditions, fairness, appropriate remuneration and career development. Efforts are also required to increase diversity within leadership levels and role holders underpinned by the Equality Act (2020), ensuring that marginalised groups are represented in senior positions and fostering professional identity across the nursing workforce. We need to ensure that policies are in place to embed the PNA role (globally), ensuring its future contribution to the development of professional identity and belonging. It is also imperative that we share the evidence of the impact of the PNA role so that this may be used by nurses globally to inform methods to support nurses in practice.

CONCLUSION

Nurse identity develops through education, clinical practice and ongoing professional growth. Challenges to belonging and identity include transitions, work dynamics and cultural barriers. Fostering a strong sense of identity has many benefits, such as influencing job satisfaction and performance, resulting in fewer vacancies, improved staff retention and higher quality care. Building nurse belonging and identity is a collaborative effort between nurses and organisations. Public perceptions of nursing also need to be addressed. By addressing challenges and providing consistent support, we can enable nurses to thrive, benefiting both patients and the healthcare system. The NHS in the United Kingdom is facing the most challenging period since it was created, and nurses are its most important asset. Investment in workforce retention and roles to support well-being and retention, such as the PNA, is imperative.

REFERENCES

Aldosari, N., Pryjmachuk, S., and Cooke, H. (2020). Newly qualified nurses' transition from learning to doing: a scoping review. *International Journal of Nursing Studies* 113: 103792. https://doi.org/10.1016/j.ijnurstu.2020.103792. Epub 2020 Oct 13. PMID: 33120135.

Allen, K.A., Kern, M.L., Rozek, C.S. et al. (2021). Belonging: a review of conceptual issues, an integrative framework, and directions for future research. *Australian Journal of Psychology* 73 (1): 87–102. https://doi.org/10.1080/00049530.2021.1883409. Epub Apr 30. PMID: 33958811; PMCID: PMC8095671.

Ariss, S.M., Earley, V., Jokhi, R., and Merodoulaki, M. (2017). *Final Evaluation Report: Pilot for New Model of Midwifery Supervision*. London: NHS England.

Austin, C. and Halpin, Y. (2021). Evaluation of a personal professional mentor scheme for newly qualified nurses. *British Journal of Nursing* 30 (11): 672–676. https://doi.org/10.12968/bjon.2021.30.11.672.

Baharum, H., Ismail, A., McKenna, L. et al. (2023). Success factors in adaptation of newly graduated nurses: a scoping review. *BioMed Central Nursing* 22: 125. https://doi.org/10.1186/s12912-023-01300-1.

Benner, P. (1984). *From Novice to Expert: Excellence and Power in Clinical Nursing Practice*. Menlo Park, CA: Addison-Wesley.

Bodey, D. (2024). Fostering belongingness: strategies to enhance learner retention in NHS healthcare education. *British Journal of Nursing* 33 (6): 312–313.

Bond, S., Merriman, C., and Walthall, H. (2020). The experiences of international nurses and midwives transitioning to work in the UK: a qualitative synthesis of the literature from 2010 to 2019. *International Journal of Nursing Studies* 110: 103693.

Boniol, M., Kunjumen, T., Nair, T.S., et al. (2022). The global health workforce stock and distribution in 2020 and 2030: a threat to equity and 'universal' health coverage? *BMJ Global Health* 7:e009316.

Buchan, J. and Catton, H. (2023). Recover to rebuild workforce for health systems effectiveness. *International Council of Nurses*. https://www.icn.ch/news/icn-report-says-shortage-nurses-global-health-emergency (accessed 19 March 2024).

Buchan, J., Charlesworth, A., Gershlick, B., and Seccombe, I.J. (2019). *A Critical Moment: NHS Staffing Trends, Retention and Attrition*. Health Foundation.

Chang Chiu A, Jermaine Monk, Maria Docal, Nancy R. Reynolds (2024) Nursing nurses: fostering safety and belonging for successful workplace assimilation of displaced nurses from war and conflict, Volume 22, Issue 2, Pages 146–152

Clarke, J., van der Riet, P., and Bowen, L. (2020). Nurses and undergraduate student nurses' experiences in collaborative clinical placement programs in acute hospitals: an integrative literature review. *Nurse Education Today* 95: 104578. https://doi.org/10.1016/j.nedt.2020.104578.

Collard, S., Scammell, J., and Tee, S. (2020). Closing the gap on nurse retention: a scoping review of implications for undergraduate education. *Nurse Education Today* 84: 104253. https://www.sciencedirect.com/science/article/pii/S0260691719306288.

Confederation NHS (2022). BME Leadership Network Shattered hopes black and minority ethnic leaders' experiences of breaking the glass ceiling in the NHS.

Craig, L. and Machin, A. (2020). Developing and sustaining nurses' service improvement capability: a phenomenological study. *British Journal of Nursing* 29 (11): 618–626.

Cummins, T. (2009). Migrant nurses' perceptions and attitudes of integration into the perioperative setting. *Journal of Advanced Nursing* 65 (8): 1611–1616.

Dahl, K., Nortvedt, L., Schrøder, J., and Bjørnnes, A.K. (2022). Internationally educated nurses and resilience: a systematic literature review. *International Nursing Review* 69 (3): 405–415. https://doi.org/10.1111/inr.12787. Epub 2022 Jul 22. PMID: 35868023; PMCID: PMC9545834.

Davda, L.S., Gallagher, J.E., and Radford, D.R. (2018). Migration motives and integration of international human resources of health in the United Kingdom: systematic review and meta-synthesis of qualitative studies using framework analysis. *Human Resources for Health* 16 (1): 27. https://doi.org/10.1186/s12960-018-0293-9. PMID: 29945616; PMCID: PMC6020357.

Deci, E.L. and Ryan, R.M. (1985). *Intrinsic Motivation and Self-determination in Human Behaviour*. Plenum.

Department of Health and Social Care (2025). 10 year health plan for England: fit for the future. https://www.gov.uk/government/publications/10-year-health-plan-for-england-fit-for-the-future (accessed 6 August 2025).

Drennan, V.M. and Ross, F. (2019). Global nurse shortages – the facts, the impact and action for change. *British Medical Bulletin* 130 (1): 25–37. https://doi.org/10.1093/bmb/ldz014.

Equality Act 2010 (2020). c39. Available at www.legislation.gov.uk/ukpga/2010/15/contents (accessed 28 January 2021).

Frangieh, J., Hughes, V., Edwards-Capello, A. et al. (2024). Fostering belonging and social connectedness in nursing: evidence-based strategies: a discussion paper for nurse students, faculty, leaders, and clinical nurses. *Nursing Outlook* 72 (4): 102174.

Garcia, R. and Qureshi, R. (2024). Nurse identity: the misrepresentation of nursing in the media. *Evidence Based Nursing* 27 (1): https://ebn.bmj.com/content/ebnurs/27/1/4.full.pdf.

Griffiths, K. (2022). Using restorative supervision to help nurses during the Covid-19 pandemic. *Nursing Times* 118 (3): 33–36.

Hawkins, N., Jeong, S., and Smith, T. (2018). Coming ready or not! An integrative review examining new graduate nurses' transition in acute care. *International Journal of Nursing Practice* 25 (3): e12714. https://doi.org/10.1111/ijn.12714.

Health and Social Care Select Committee (2022). Third Special Report – Expert Panel: Evaluation of Government's Commitments in the Area of the Health and Social Care Workforce in England.

Health Education England (2020). Growing Nursing Numbers Literature Review on Nurses Leaving the NHS.

Health Foundation (2019). What happens when you make nursing a more attractive profession? www.health.org.uk/features-and-opinion/features/what-happens-when-you-make-nursing-a-more-attractive-profession (accessed 24 December 2025).

Hill, B. (2023). Professional identity in nursing. *British Journal of Nursing* 32 (15): 706.

Hill, B. (2024). The importance of belongingness and friendship within the nursing community. *The British Journal of Nursing* 33 (6): https://www.britishjournalofnursing.com/content/regulars/the-importance-of-belongingness-and-friendships-within-the-nursing-community.

Hinkley, T.-L., Strouse, S.M., and Butcher, D. (Terri)(2023). Professional identity in nursing: the role of efficacy in navigating the work environment. *Nurse Leader* 21 (2): 174–178.

Hirata, H. and Harvath, T.A. (2016). Japanese care workers' perception of dementia-related physically and psychologically aggressive behaviour symptoms. *International Journal of Older People Nursing* 12 (1): e12119.

Ho, P. (2025). Professional identity among nursing students: a longitudinal analysis of student experiences and developmental pathways. *Journal of Professional Nursing* 58: 104–111. https://doi.org/10.1016/j.profnurs.2025.03.009.

Ho, S., Stonehouse, R., and Snowden, A. (2021). 'It was quite a shock': a qualitative study of the impact of organisational and personal factors on newly qualified nurses. *Journal of Clinical Nursing* 30: 2373–2385.

Hogan, M. (2023). The role of the professional nurse advocate: improving both staff and patient safety. https://www.pslhub.org/learn/professionalising-patient-safety/training/staff-clinical/the-role-of-the-professional-nurse-advocate-improving-both-staff-and-patient-safety-r9373 (accessed 24 December 2025).

International Council of Nurses. (2020). Nursing definitions. https://www.icn.ch/nursing-policy/nursing-definitions (accessed 24 December 2025).

Jenkins, C. and Smythe, A. (2024). 'What are nurses' and healthcare workers' cultural understandings of dementia?' An integrative literature review.

Dementia 24 (3): 552–576. https://journals.sagepub.com/doi/full/10.1177/14713012241285525.

John, S. (2019). Imposter syndrome: why some of us doubt our competence. *Nursing Times [online]* 115 (2): 23–24.

Kamau S, Koskenranta M, Isakov TM, Kuivila H, Oikarainen A, Tomietto M, Mikkonen K. Culturally and linguistically diverse registered nurses' experiences of integration into nursing workforce - A qualitative descriptive study. *Nurse Education Today* 2023 Feb;121:105700. doi: https://doi.org/10.1016/j.nedt.2022.105700

Kelly, E., Stoye, G., and Warner, M. (2002). *Factors Associated with Staff Retention in the NHS Acute Sector*. The Institute for Fiscal Studies.

Kings Fund (2024). The King's Fund responds to the Nursing and Midwifery Council's annual data registration report. www.kingsfund.org.uk/insight-and-analysis/press-releases/nursing-midwifery-data-registration-report?utm_source=chatgpt.com (accessed 6 August 2024).

Laing D and Smythe A (2024) The challenges for nurses assimilating to new health care systems. *Journal of International Nurses.* 72(1):e13078. doi: https://doi.org/10.1111/inr.13078. PMID: 39690509

Lanada, J.A. and Culligan, K. (2024). The experiences of internationally educated nurses who joined the workforce in England. *British Journal of Nursing* 33: 2. https://www.britishjournalofnursing.com/content/professional/the-experiences-of-internationally-educated-nurses-who-joined-the-nursing-workforce-in-england.

Lee, E. and De Gagne, J.C. (2022). The impact of resilience on turnover among newly graduated nurses: a 1-year follow-up study. *Journal of Nursing Management* 30 (5): https://doi.org/10.1111/jonm.13613.

Lees-Deutsch, L., Adegboye, A., Bayes, N. et al. (2023). *National Evaluation of the Professional Nurse Advocate Programme: SUSTAIN – Supervision, Support, Advocacy for Improvement in Nursing, Mixed Methods Study.* Coventry University.

Lees-Deutsch, L., Palmer, S., Adegboye, A. et al. (2025). Professional nurse advocates: a national evaluation survey of the programme in England. *BioMed Central Nursing* http://doi.org/10.1186/s12912-025-03415-z.

López-Verdugo, M., Ponce-Blandón, J.A., López-Narbona, F.J. et al. (2021). Social image of nursing. An integrative review about a yet unknown profession. *Nursing Reports* 11 (2): 460–474. https://doi.org/10.3390/nursrep11020043. PMID: 34968221; PMCID: PMC8608107.

Mansour, M. and Mattukoyya, R. (2019). Development of assertive communication skills in nursing preceptorship programmes: a qualitative insight from newly qualified nurses. *Nursing Management* 26 (4): 29–35. https://doi.org/10.7748/nm.2019.e1857.

Mazzocco, K., Petitti, D.B., Fong, K.T. et al. (2009). Surgical team behaviors and patient outcomes. *American Journal of Surgery* 197: 678–685.

Mohammed, S., Peter, E., Killackey, T., and Maciver, J. (2018). The "nurse as hero" discourse in the COVID-19 pandemic: a poststructural discourse analysis. *International Journal of Nursing Studies* 117: 103887. https://doi.org/10.1016/j.ijnurstu.2021.103887. Epub 2021 Jan 26. PMID: 33556905; PMCID: PMC9749900.Nursing and Midwifery Council. The Code www.nmc.org.uk/standards/code.

Ndirangu, E.W., Sarki, A.M., Mbekenga, C., and Edwards, G. (2024). Professional image of nursing and midwifery in East Africa: an exploratory analysis. *BioMed Central Nursing* 20 (1): 37. https://doi.org/10.1186/s12912-020-00531-w. PMID: 33676509; PMCID: PMC7936462.

NHS Digital (2018). NHS workforce statistics – December 2018 (Including supplementary information on mental health workforce. https://digital.nhs.uk/data-and-information/publications/statistical/nhs-workforce-statistics/december-2018

NHS Digital (2023). NHS workforce statistics – December 2022 (Including selected provisional statistics for January 2023) [Delayed from 30/03/23]: NHS England. https://digital.nhs.uk/data-andinformation/publications/statistical/nhs-workforce-statistics/december-2022

NHS England (2021). The promise. https://www.england.nhs.uk/our-nhs-people/online-version/lfaop/our-nhs-people-promise/the-promise (accessed 6 August 2025).

NHS England (2023a). HS equality, diversity, and inclusion improvement plan. https://www.england.nhs.uk/long-read/nhs-equality-diversity-and-inclusion-improvement-plan (accessed 24 December 2025).

NHS England (2023b). New figures show NHS workforce most diverse it has ever been. https://www.england.nhs.uk/2023/02/new-figures-show-nhs-workforce-most-diverse-it-has-ever-been (accessed 7 August 2023).

NHS England (2023c). NHS long term workforce plan brief guide from NHS England – June 2023. *Nurse Leader* 22 (2): 146–152.

NHS England (2025). Staff leaving the NHS among lowest in over a decade. https://www.england.nhs.uk/north-west/2025/03/04/staff-leaving-the-nhs-among-lowest-in-over-a-decade/?utm_source=chatgpt.com (accessed 6 August 2025)

Patel, E., Varghese, J., and Hamm, K. (2024). Defining sense of belonging in nursing – an evolutionary concept analysis. *Journal of Professional Nursing* 54: 151–163.

Pearce, L. (2023). Take the lead in a nurse advocate role: professional nurse advocates give clinical and well-being support to colleagues, in a role underpinned by new education. *Nursing Standard* 38 (8): 55–56.

Peters, A., Palomo, R., and Pittet, D. (2020). The great nursing brain drain and its effects on patient safety. *Antimicrobial Resistance and Infection Control* 9: 57. https://doi.org/10.1186/s13756-020-00719-4.

Poorchangizi, B., Farokhzadian, J., Abbaszadeh, A. et al. (2017). The importance of professional values from clinical nurses' perspective in hospitals of a medical university in Iran. *BioMed Central Medical Ethics* 18 (1): 20. https://doi.org/10.1186/s12910-017-0178-9. PMID: 28249603; PMCID: PMC5333397.

Pressley, C., Newton, D., Garside, J. et al. (2022). Global migration and factors that support acculturation and retention of international nurses: a systematic review. *International Journal of Nursing Studies Advances* 4: 100083. ISSN 2666-142X. https://doi.org/10.1016/j.ijnsa.2022.100083.

Pung, L.X. and Goh, Y.S. (2017). Challenges faced by international nurses when migrating: an integrative literature review. *International Nursing Review* 64 (1): 146–165.

Reinhardt AC, León TG, Amatya A. Why nurses stay: analysis of the registered nurse workforce and the relationship to work environments. *Applied Nursing Research* 2020 Oct;55:151316. doi: https://doi.org/10.1016/j.apnr.2020.151316

Roth, C., Berger, S., Krug, K. et al. (2021). Internationally trained nurses and host nurses' perceptions of safety culture, work-life-balance, burnout, and job demand during workplace integration: a cross-sectional study. *BioMed Central Nursing* 20 (1): 77. https://doi.org/10.1186/s12912-021-00581-8. PMID: 33993868; PMCID: PMC8127287.

Sabancıogullari, S. and Dogan, S. (2015). Effects of the professional identity development programme on the professional identity, job satisfaction and burnout levels of nurses: a pilot study. *International Journal of Nursing Practice* 21: 847–857.

Shen, J., Yu, X., Bolstad, A. et al. (2012). Effects of a short-term linguistic class on communication competence of international nurses. *Nursing Economics* 30 (1): 21–28.

Smythe, A. and Carter, V. (2022). The experiences and perceptions of newly qualified nurses in the UK: an integrative literature review. *Nurse Education in Practice* 62: 103338. ISSN 1471-5953.

Smythe, A. Walker, W., and Flatt C. (2023). The role of the professional nurse advocate and A-EQUIP model in practice: a qualitative exploratory study. Final report submitted to NHS England and NHS Improvement, June 2023. https://future.nhs.uk/ProfessionalNurseAdvocate/view?objectId=177377541

Squire, D., Gonzalez, L., and Shayan, C. (2024). Enhancing sense of belonging in nursing student clinical placements to advance learning and identity development. *Journal of Professional Nursing* 51: 109–114. ISSN 8755-7223.

UNHCR (2023). The UN Refugee Agency. *Global Trends Report 2022*. https://www.unhcr.org/global-trends-report-2022 (accessed 11 November 2023).

Van der Cingel, M. and Brouwer, J. (2021). What makes a nurse today? A debate on the nursing professional identity and its need for change. *Nursing Philosophy* 22 (2): e12343. https://doi.org/10.1111/nup.12343. Epub 2021 Jan 15. PMID: 33450124.

Wade, R. (2023). Embedding the A-EQUIP model of restorative supervision in a critical care unit by professional nurse advocates. *British Journal of Nursing* 32 (15): 744–747.

West, M., Bailey, S., Williams, E. et al. (2020). The courage of compassion: supporting nurses and midwives to deliver high-quality care. *The Kings Fund* https://assets.kingsfund.org.uk/f/256914/x/ccc7dc0553/courage_of_compassion_summary_2020.pdf.

Woldasemayat, Y.L., Mekonnen Zeru, L., and Demissie, A.A. (2022). Perception towards nursing profession and associated factors among patients at Jimma Medical Center, Ethiopia. A cross-sectional study. *International Journal of Africa Nursing Sciences* 17: 100445.

Zizzo, K.A. and Xu, Y. (2009). Post-hire transitional programs for international nurses: a systematic review. *Journal of Continuing Education in Nursing* 40 (2): 57–64, 65–66. https://doi.org/10.3928/00220124-20090201-02. PMID: 19263926.

CHAPTER 3

Leadership Models and the PNA Role

Jill Barr

Coventry University Health and Care, Coventry, UK, London, UK

Learning Points

1. Identify the evolution of a range of leadership theories
2. Compare and contrast the various leadership theories
3. Critically discuss the application of these theories in relation to the PNA role

HISTORICAL CONTEXT

Historically, midwifery led the way in clinical supervision from the first Midwives Act (1902), where all midwives had a midwifery supervisor to oversee practice as they had independent practice status but within defined limits. Nationally, the midwifery supervision model, enshrined in statute, was variable, but in 1974, it became practice to appoint senior midwifery managers as supervisors (Williams and Hunt 1996; Henshaw et al. 2013. There were compromises and conflicts with the early supervision model, but the benefits for women, families, midwives and midwifery were seen to be generally positive. In 2017, which followed the Short Report (1980) and Changing Childbirth (DOH 1993), a new model of midwifery clinical supervision was launched and set out plans for the transition from a statutory model of supervision to an employer-led professional model (NHS England 2017) called A-EQUIP using Professional Midwifery Advocates (PMAs).

Health visiting became the next focus for clinical supervision, and it was recognised that these HCPs were facing huge challenges in practice as populations diversified, and child and family health were becoming very complex, and as lone family health visitors, they noted the stress of the role and often felt unsupported. Wallbank and Woods (2012) highlighted the concern for children and the drive to encompass the new Solihull approach and new skills for family motivational interviewing. 'Restorative Clinical Supervision' (RCS) was launched and was eventually commissioned to support the role leading up to the Health Visiting Implementation Plan in 2011. They also noted that RCS was essential to increase job satisfaction, vitality, reduce stress and emotional exhaustion of the role. The aim was to increase the resilience of health visitors so that they can act on risk and improve service quality as well as increase sensitivity towards themselves and the families they care for. Wallbank and Woods (2013) also noted the value of restorative supervision in helping health visitors to reclaim their role autonomy and strong clinical leadership to deal with the complexity of hard-to-help families and safeguarding children.

Nursing, Management and Leadership Theories

Through the lens of nursing practice, the PNA role development is relatively new, and yet, the value of leadership, management and supervisory support was seen to be an essential focus during the COVID-19 epidemic. National health policy required senior hospital nurses to lead the PNA initiative, with the initial priority on supporting nurses in intensive and critical care units. Formal clinical supervision in nursing was not always transparent, as the many forms of nursing practice required different models to address practitioner needs. The changing nature of nursing however was a driver to value how clinical supervision as a formal leadership process led to improved patient care and service quality, particularly during COVID (Baldwin et al. 2022). Mentoring, supporting, monitoring and learning were seen as key elements, but care generally was regarded as a hierarchical process.

ACTIVITY

Q: What is it about nursing that the PNA and restorative clinical supervision aim to address?

A: This is really supervisee-driven and so topics may be wide-ranging. For instance, it may concern a new coronary care unit (CCU) nurse's anxieties about growing confident using the unit technology.

More experienced staff in this area may be concerned with dealing with end-of-life care/bereavement counselling skills, infection control and any reflective account where they need support. They may require support in dealing with the stress of any critical work situation or a recent conflict involving family members. However, it may also be of a more personal nature regarding family health, financial stress or domestic relationships where they need a supportive listener. The PNA therefore needs to consider using their leadership skills to determine how to 'manage' the variety of staff needs.

Trait Theory and PNA Role

The 'Great Man' theory was popularised around the 1900s and focused on the idea of some universal traits of leaders. The 'Great Man' theory is based on the belief that leaders possess exceptional qualities. It has been argued that this theory was born out of the philosophy of Aristotle (384–322 BC) who believed that some are *born to lead,* and others are *born to be led,* thus linking back to the notion of leadership and followership. It also raises the assumption that some people have specific leadership qualities and others do not. This assumption may be seen to identify potential leaders for the future. Biased towards the leadership in the military and thus reflecting masculine traits for successful campaigns in the armed forces, it is argued whether this theory is still of value. 'Trait' theory is still transparent when job descriptions and person specifications are the basis for suitable qualities when shortlisting candidates for posts. NHS England (2017) produced a person specification for the new PMA role. The RCN (2023) produced professional PNA education and training standards and mapped these against the NMC (2018a) Code, the education framework (NMC (2018b) as well as the NMC

Proficiencies and Standards (NMC 2018c). It was also aligned to the Framework for Higher Education of UK Degree-Awarding Bodies. In section 1 of the RCN document, selection criteria are laid down to apply to take on the post-graduate education/training for the PNA role. This is one example of how leadership is manifesting the trait theory linked to the role.

Bennis (1999) highlighted that past research showed that there were seven attributes essential to leadership:

1. Technical competence in one's own field
2. Conceptual, abstract or strategic thinking
3. Track record
4. People skills
5. Taste to cultivate talent
6. Judgement
7. Character

More recently, Covey (2004) also noted traits regarding the seven habits of highly effective people, and although not specifically linked to leadership, desirable PNA traits could be reflected.

1. Be proactive
2. Begin with the end in mind
3. Put first things first
4. Think win-win
5. Seek to understand first before making yourself understood
6. Learn to synergise
7. Sharpen the saw

ACTIVITY

Q: Do you think effective PNA roles align with any of these traits suggested above? What other traits are seen as valuable today?

A: You may agree or disagree but think the following are useful traits from Covey's list of 'habits'.

- They initiate action prior to incidents and get things done rather than react to incidents.

- They focus on patient and staff satisfaction as an end result.
- They have a good prioritisation agenda.
- They think about trying to get a solution to please most/all stakeholders.
- They are good communicators, putting listening (to staff concerns) as a priority.
- Rather than getting their own concerns over to staff to understand wider perspectives. They focus on bringing agreed change to meet.
- They work together with a number of disciplines and ranks to find good solutions to problems/issues.
- They work at improving and motivating themselves towards a good work and life balance.

You may have found the above question difficult, as the way people lead others varies in time and place; sometimes it is hard to identify characteristics that they all share. This may be because in different contexts, leaders require different attributes. You are not alone in such difficulties. The literature is still confusing, and there is much debate about the value of trait theory in the world of work today. Trait theory has been challenged as the research was found to be inconclusive and contradictory, especially as the relationship between leaders/teams and the context of the situation was seen as more important. Leadership traits seem to become more noticeable in retrospect, alongside recognition of significant achievements.

ACTIVITY

Can you jot down what you consider your own specific nursing traits, skills, talents or abilities are and see if they link to any of the above ideas?

Case Study

Pat as a senior NHS Trust PNA lead characterised these traits. Although not a PNA herself, she was keen to provide a culture where top-down and bottom-up strategies and open communication were valued and facilitated to allow 8 hours of protected time for PNA RCS activity. She set up some

'Shared decision-making' [SDM] Councils to facilitate the growth of the initiative and has plans to strengthen a PNA buddy system. Pat is proud of the Trust, which has 'Magnet' status (US-based); thus, there is a noted 'Pathway to Excellence' culture – finding out things that work less well: making it happen. She believes that it is important to have commitment from the top of the Trust [Board members] and value the 8 hours per month of protected time for PNA activity, securing SDM and meeting spaces for staff. She is involved in Nursing and Midwifery Education Tariff (NMET) forums and the local PNA Steering group to recruit for the PNA training and manages the funded places for the Master's level module, as well as investing in 'Continuing Professional Development' (CPD) activity. Some of the challenges involve the staff challenges studying at level 7 and PNA staff targets, as well as the need to address the NHS England requirements for monthly reports. She also recognises that other staff groups could benefit from RCS and hopes to expand and make the project more equitable for other health care professionals (HCPs) and balance the gender differences. It was recognisable that she was an excellent listener and the importance of trying to understand those in PNA roles in making a difference, rather than sending out top-down e-mails of expectations and micromanage staff was clear.

ACTIVITY

Q: How does this case study reflect Laschinger et al.'s (2010) Empowerment Model?

A: You may want to reflect on the access to information, support, resources, learning and development, as well as formal and informal power elements for PNAs to consider.

Bureaucracy, Management and Leadership Theories

The early 'Scientific Management' era was connected with similar models of industrial management and concerned bureaucratic operations where power and control were seen as the best way of managing staff in a hierarchical structure to make production effective and efficient. Bureaucracy was defined by Weber (1921) and is seen as a way for a clear hierarchy and division of labour. In terms of the health industry, this equated with greater patient throughput or timely service episodes. One of the key features of our National Health Service (NHS) is that it is seen as one of the most bureaucratic organisations in Britain and even Europe. Dickinson et al. (2017) related the work of Mintzberg (1998) as both described the NHS as a 'professional bureaucracy'. Policies, procedures, standards and targets characterise the nature of the bureaucracy and transnationalism. These management and leadership theories still relate to social functionalism and concern how social organisation is maintained and how it functions in today's health industry.

Case Study

Lily is a dedicated CCU (Band 6) nurse with a 30-hour week contract and is keen to support her colleagues in their challenging clinical roles as an appointed PNA in order to improve the service and support staff. She has been given a number of hours for the PNA role, but feels she is not only expected to manage RCS for a number of band 5 nurses who are struggling to cope with their own self/family health issues as well as listen to a physiotherapist and junior doctor on an ad hoc basis affected by a series of unexpected deaths. The other aspect of the role requires Lily to submit the data required by the NHS England.

She needs to submit the monthly data returns to her PNA Lead on:

- How many specific individual RCS sessions held
- How many group sessions held and how many individuals in total were present
- How many education and development sessions held – following incident reports, errors and complaints
- How many new improvement projects/programmes were supported by PNAs
- How many new career conversations held (revalidation and personal development)

She feels this monthly data submission often encroaches on her supervisory role and notes the stress by putting the data submission on hold. She finds the PNA meetings with the Chief Nursing and Midwifery (CNM) meetings every 3 months to discuss RCS trends and confidential issues raised, which may need escalating for helpful. The Senior Staff also have confidential weekly meetings to discuss possible common solutions.

> **Explore**
>
> - The importance and value of the bureaucracy of data required and the impact and late/non-submission of data required by Lily, PNA Leads, staff and patients/families.

Social structures, their integration, harmony and evolutionary stability in an organisation underpin scientific management and bureaucracy (Weitz et al. 2011). Fayol (1925) first identified the main management functions were 'Planning, Organising, Coordination and Control'. Daft (2017, pp. 13–14) confirmed that the five functions to managing effectively are planning, organising, staffing, directing and controlling. Ideas within this category centre on the nature and consequences of structures and how leadership as a structure supports the function of the organisation to carry out its work, with attention given to

Sources of power and influence over others

How various roles relate to the functions in an organisation to meet its needs.

The emphasis of leadership here is not on *what they have* but on *what they do*, who they *influence* and how this *relates to the function* a particular PNA plays in an organisation. The overlap of appointed leaders or managers and naturally emerging leaders could be argued that there are some similarities in the two concepts of management and leadership as well as some differences. Other relevant but older leadership theories such as the Fiedler model (1967) and and Vroom-Jago model (1988) may be worth further exploring in terms of situational and decision-making opportunities.

Case Study

Rose is a band 7 critical care senior nurse with an early PNA status since COVID in 2022.

She has regular communications with the Trust PNA lead (non-PNA trained) but feels fully supported. In a hierarchy, she has responsibility to three band 6 PNAs who in turn have responsibility for three band 5 PNAs. However, this structure involves staff from various clinical areas and thus represents a matrix of PNAs, meaning clinical staff who have a separate structure of managers and PNA support.

> **Reflect On**
>
> - Whether this PNA hierarchy may be helpful or of concern.
> - How does this PNA support structure connect with clinical management.

CONTINGENCY THEORIES

Leadership Styles

A leader's style of behaviour provides further theories on the topic. Lewin (1951) and White and Lippitt (2006) identified various types of leader behaviour. One way of looking at leadership style is in connection to the *power* that a leader exerts over staff in a team, and these can be situated on a continuum from autocratic at one end through democratic to 'Laissez-Faire' at the opposite end.

- **Autocratic or Authoritarian Style:** the leader exercises power in decision-making and controls the rewards and punishments for staff regarding compliance.
- **Democratic and Participative Style:** the leader encourages all staff to interact and to contribute to making decisions.
- **Laissez-faire Style:** the leader *conscientiously* makes the decision to pass the focus of power on to staff in a genuine laissez-faire style. This is distinct from abdication or 'non-leadership' where the 'leader' refuses to make any decisions.

A person's leadership style has a great deal of influence on the work environment. For many years, it was believed that leaders employed a consistently dominant style. It was also felt that autocracy and laissez-faire styles were less acceptable than the democratic style. Later, it was felt that there was a continuum of styles between autocratic and laissez-faire behaviours and that those leaders moved dynamically between styles in response to new situations. Tannenbaum and Schmidt (1958) highlighted that the continuum model is too simplistic that a mixture of autocracy and democracy is needed and that elements such as leadership skills, the situation and the abilities of the group are required for effective leadership. The impact of the situation on the behaviour of a leader highlighted that leadership styles of individuals *could* be changed. In essence, one can think of these theories as being quite fluid and maneuverable – an 'if/then' sort of relationship between several variables – so that *if* a certain situation arose, *then* it would be dealt with in the most appropriate manner. Within the clinical situation, we work a good deal within the confines of such theory; we rarely know what is going to happen next, so we must adapt to each situation as it occurs.

Case Study

Mo is a new PNA (grade 6) and has recently met with Helen, a newly qualified Band 5 CCU nurse who is feeling overwhelmed with her workload. He notes the importance of listening to Helen and helping her to offload her concerns. Mo makes a note to check out on a new follow-up appointment.

Recent national evaluation research into the PNA role and its impact on patient outcomes as well as personal and professional staff impact has been illuminating (Lees-Deutsch et al. 2023, 2025; Walker et al., 2025). A mixed research methodology approach was used. Nurses generally found RCS very positive in terms of Laschinger's model of

- enhancing structural empowerment,
- psychological empowerment and
- positive work feelings.

Feeling valued, supported and listened to were the over-riding perspectives. However, in the early days, nurses described their 'offloading of issues' rather than being active participants in a process leading towards greater resilience as an issue. The support of experienced nurses (PNAs) in practice helps nurses feel valued and empowered; RCS and career conversations were felt to enable nurses, who might otherwise leave the profession, to stay. The programme has opened opportunities for nurses to engage in further study and development following the programme. These factors are important in the context of a global workforce retention crisis.

Transactional and Transformational Leadership Styles

Burns (1978) noted that transactional and transformational styles were also at ends of a continuum. Transactional culture had much criticism compared with the need for a more transformational culture. However, Bass (1985) argued that they were styles that could exist beside each other and developed a framework where transformational leadership consisted of four dimensions, namely

- idealised influence,
- inspirational motivation,
- intellectual stimulation and
- individualised consideration (Bass and Avolio 1990).

The bureaucracy of the National Health Service has benefited from the contractual or transactional leadership style in stable environments in the past. The growth in policies, procedures and employment law began to develop. It was also felt that leaders and teams found mutual satisfaction within these transactional relationships by 'knowing where they stood'. Huston (2024, p. 45) identified the characteristics of a transactional leader as someone who:

focuses on management tasks

is directive and result-orientated

uses trade-offs to meet goals

does not identify shared values

examines causes

uses contingency rewards.

The emergence of Apple, Sony, MS and even Tesla electric cars transformed the business world into thinking differently about the need for creativity and changing with the times. Traditional ways of working, where employees had a job for life and were rewarded for their loyalty to the employer, were starting to disappear. More creative problem solving was required to look for new markets, new products and services and to 'fit' within the emerging global economy. This environment affected healthcare within public services. *Transformational leadership* theories started to surface, in contrast to transactional leadership theories. Transformational theories of leadership are based on the idea that leaders are people who *motivate* others to perform by encouraging them to see a vision and change their perception of reality. Such leaders are seen as committed individuals with long-term vision and a need to empower others and who are interested in the consequences. They use:

charisma

individualized consideration

intellectual stimulation to produce greater effort, effectiveness and satisfaction in followers

inspiration through symbols. (Bass and Avolio 1990)

Case Study

Paul highlights that the importance of a PNA is to educate and inform staff in a team meeting of a recent audit, discuss the results and get the team to offer up ideas on how they might have better support to achieve better outcomes.

Burns (2010) identified that the transforming process is one in which leaders and followers raise each other to higher levels of morals and motivation. Hence, values such as liberty, peace, equality and humanitarianism are often emphasised, rather than values based on individual benefits. However, it has been noted that transformational leaders can have the potential for accruing a good deal of control and power, which can lead to the exploitation of large numbers of followers.

ACTIVITY

Q: What are your thoughts on becoming a qualified PNA?

A: You may have thought about expanding your skills of leadership, counselling and clinical practice. These will surely relate to your NMC (2018d) Standards of Proficiency on many platforms outlined. Do check these out if you are a UK nurse or midwife.

Adair 'Action – Centred' Leadership

Adair's action leadership model (2010, p. 24) focused on the interacting spheres of addressing the required work tasks, the needs of the working team and the needs of individual people. This complex leadership role involves how leaders have to compromise the various activities associated with each sphere. In terms of connecting the functions of the organisation to the people, Adair (2010, p. 24) uses the idea of 'action-centred leadership' where the group leader, to be seen as effective, needs to have the ability to meet three functions:

to achieve the required role task(s)

to address the needs of individual team members

to maintain the team

ACTIVITY

Q: How might Adair's model of leadership apply in the PNA role?

A: PNAs supporting clinical practitioners fit with this simple model. When exploring patient care, the

- **Task Needs**: Relate to planning and meeting relevant clinical staff and completing monthly audit
- **Individual Needs:** Relates to offering individual support to help address their needs.
- **Team Maintenance:** Concerns other PNAs, attending management meeting (shared decision-making) and effectively managing time

---

Case Study

PNA Lizzie raises a difficult issue of a recent ward medication error with her supervisees on an individual basis and asking them to reflect on the episode, checking on the patients, relatives and staff. She tries to identify the learning points from this and disseminating them so that others can learn. Supporting the staff members through this and seeing everyone's perspective on the issues can be seen as helpful.

HUMAN RELATIONS MANAGEMENT

These theories emerged around the 1970s and 1980s and influenced the humanistic view of leadership as opposed to 'hard' management and the importance of people over productivity became popular. The theories that emerged within this category focused initially on how leaders behaved towards their team, but later, the importance of the effects of team behaviour *on leadership* was realised.

Herzberg's (1966) 'Two Factor Motivation Theory' was an example of *hedonic or pleasure* theories where praise underpins the way people behave. Herzberg discovered from his research that certain factors are related to job satisfaction or dissatisfaction. These were *not* opposites of each other. Trying to address dissatisfaction factors would not lead to satisfaction. If you want to lead and motivate a team towards improved performance, you need to eliminate job dissatisfaction and then focus on the satisfaction factors:

Factors for Satisfaction – 'Motivating' Factors

Achievement

Recognition

The work itself

Advancement

Growth

Factors for Dissatisfaction – 'Hygiene' Factors

Company policies

Supervision

Relationship with supervisor and peers

Work conditions

Status

Security

<table>
<tr><td>Case Study</td></tr>
<tr><td>Patience, a band 6 PNA, provides some advice regarding an upcoming band 6 interview for James, explaining the process, the scoring matrix, Trust values and tips. She further encourages him by raising recent short courses he has taken and then offers to help with a mock interview for practice.</td></tr>
</table>

Traditional management and leadership theories started to be questioned, particularly in the UK health industry, which had grown more complex and required more staff resilience and adaptability so that newer ideas were forming. Kouzes and Posner (2007) focused on leadership as a human relationship and noted the five exemplary practices of leadership:

- Model the way
- Inspire a shared vision
- Challenge the process
- Enable others to act
- Encourage the heart

Leadership Theories to Form Organisational Culture

Organisational culture formation and leadership are entwined (Schein 1985). Transactional culture and transformational culture have been differentiated as being part of organisational life. Leadership has thus emerged in the context of changing cultures and dynamics, which is especially important within different healthcare environments, even within the NHS. Schein (1992, p. 237) defined organisational culture as:

> *The pattern of basic assumptions that a given group has invented, discovered or developed in learning to cope with its problems of external adaptation and internal integration and therefore taught to new members as the correct way to perceive, think and feel in relation to those problems.*

He felt that leadership needs to be seen in a cultural context. The type of leadership required in healthcare is therefore one that fits with the culture of the organisation where health services are delivered. A number of theoretical models regarding organisational culture have been developed and are still relevant, which may be useful to review (Handy 1985; Schein 1992; Johnson and Scholes 1989).

Daft (2017, p. 11) indicates that the *humble* leader is now more likely to succeed than the *charismatic hero* leader of yesterday. West (2024) goes further and highlights the valued role of the compassionate leader using the four elements of compassion:

- Paying attention to the other, being present and noticing their suffering – *attending*
- Understanding what is causing the others distress, by making an appraisal of the cause, ideally through listening to dialogue with that person to achieve a shared understanding – *understanding*
- Having an empathetic response, mirroring the other's feelings, having a felt relation with the other's distress without being overwhelmed by those feelings – *empathising*
- Taking intelligent (thoughtful, wise and appropriate) action to help relieve the others suffering – *helping*

NEW LEADERSHIP

Barr and Dowding (2026, p. 78) noted that in the 1980s and 1990s, Rosebeth Kanter, a Harvard professor and nurse researcher, developed the theory of structural power in organisations. In complex health organisations, some staff may feel insignificant and powerless to make improvement changes.

In terms of nursing, there has also been a historical feature of feeling in the role of the 'doctors handmaiden', and globally, this may still hold true.

As new roles have been steadily developing in the health service amidst a shortage of doctors and nurses, we see an expansion/extension of nursing roles and nurse prescribers, nurse consultants, community matrons' roles developed. Nurse leaders need to be think about their personal and organisational abilities in the following areas:

- Self-mastery
- Strategic planning
- Continual learning
- Creator of partnerships
- Team facilitator

Kanter (1983) opined that a leader's power will grow by sharing the power through empowering others, and as a result, leaders will realise increased organisational performance (Fox 1998). Furthermore, Kanter posits that with tools, information, and support, people's skill base will improve, they will increasingly make informed decisions and overall accomplish more, thereby benefiting the organisation as a whole (Fox 1998). Formal power is that which accompanies high-visibility jobs and requires a primary focus on independent decision-making. Informal power comes from building relationships and alliances with peers and colleagues (Wagner et al. 2019). By providing this to staff, it has been found that there is increased job satisfaction, commitment, trust and a marked decrease in job burnout. Kantor's theory has proven to have a measurable impact on both staff empowerment and greater peer cohesion, support from supervisors, and staff autonomy grew (Krebs et al. 2008). Thus, from this, it has been found that there is increased job satisfaction, commitment, trust and a marked decrease in job burnout.

Kanter's theory still resonates as one of the most basic frameworks to guide practice in order to improve organisational efficacy. Where healthcare leaders have been able to put into practice empowerment models, i.e. Magnet Hospitals, there has been success within challenging times (Krebs et al. 2008). It was also found that staff retention rates of healthcare professionals improve when empowerment principles are put into place. Laschinger (2010) used this work of Kanter to further link empowerment of health professionals to the empowerment of the patient for better health outcomes and devised an 'Empowerment Model', incorporating structural power, psychological empowerment and positive feelings at work.

In concurring with these views, Mintzberg (1998, p. 588) highlighted the importance of vision, shared ideals, the creation of organisational pride, developing environments for energies and innovation as essential attributes of leadership. He also identified that a unique and essential leadership function is to build an organisation's culture and shape its evolution. Personal mastery, group synergy, learning and sustainable development of new leadership theory started to emerge (Bennis et al. 1994; Malby 1994). Scott (1998) pointed to the value of improving relationships between settings, process-based skills and professional judgement for the future of clinical leadership and identifies that the time is right for leading in this way within a framework of increased accountability. Daft (2017, p. 15) has noted that this new leadership era focuses on the need for leaders to show subtler personal qualities that are not transparent but are powerful, such as enthusiasm, integrity, courage and humility. He identifies that *management* encourages emotional distance, whereas *leadership* requires emotional connectivity.

Case Study

Chris, a junior RN, complained regularly and could be particularly disruptive to new staff or students, and the team felt that he was overly negative. As a PNA, I listened to his venting and frustration. At the end of our session, we agreed on two points with easy practical solutions that could be implemented easily. A couple of months later, Chris approached me for another supervision session and shared how powerful the first session had been, realising that some things couldn't be changed, but valued the changes made positively. I recognised two things: he needed a safe space to talk things out, and daily frustrations were minimised. Second, the team changed their view of Chris and his improvement suggestions benefitted everyone, and he was credited with suggesting the changes that worked.

AUTHENTIC, ETHICAL AND VALUE-BASED LEADERSHIP

Authentic leadership is a relatively new leadership idea. Northouse (2016, pp. 195–223) infers that its focus is on genuineness and a moral link between leaders and followers and that it concerns intrapersonal perspectives or processes. It is felt that authentic leadership develops over time and is influenced by personal life events. Avolio and Gardner (2005, p. 318) identified that their authentic leadership model focused on values, identity, emotions, goals and motives, along with follower trust, engagement and well-being, sustainable outcomes.

George (2003) identified five characteristics of 'Authentic' leaders

- a sense of purpose and passion
- a set of moral values and behaviours
- a belief in relationships and connectedness
- a sense of self-discipline and consistency
- compassion and 'heart'.

Case Study

Rina is a newly recruited international nurse working on a medical ward and is very upset about an experience with an elderly patient the previous day. The patient shouted at her when she offered to help him to the toilet. He used racist comments and asked her to go and get an English nurse to help him. How do you think the PNA should manage to support this member of staff? What are the ethical issues to consider? Can you think about other topics that PNAs would help staff with?

Some other topics that PNAs listen to relate to the personal worries of staff. For example, children who are ill, financial issues, domestic violence and even the impact of the menopause so wide and varying. Authentic leaders are seen as being important in helping colleagues find significance and positive association at work so that they can deal with their novel, chaotic and vigorously altering work surroundings, and such leaders are essential in organisations today. On the other hand, there needs to be more research into the validity of this model as it is still so new and focuses on positive higher-order characteristics, which may be difficult to measure (Northouse 2016, p. 208). Mubarak and Noor (2018) used research to explore the relationship that exists between authentic leadership and employee creativity in project-based organisations. They found that employee creativity is significantly associated with authentic leadership, work engagement and psychological empowerment. They also revealed that extra-engaged employees at work were more creative and had a sense of empowerment affected by the relationship between authentic leadership and employee creativity. Creativity is needed in the health service, but a compromise needs to be made as there can be too much creative change. Harris and Mayo (2018, p. 611) noted that ethical leadership qualities and behaviours are encouraged by the UK Care Quality Commission (CQC), which has stressed the necessity for good leadership in healthcare and stated that this is characterised by, among other things, strength and transparency, and an openness to challenge and change.

SYSTEMS AND GLOBAL LEADERSHIP

Post-heroic transformational leadership theories focus on the necessity of change and encourage the change process to originate from engaged team members at *all levels* of the organisation (Alimo-Metcalfe and Alban-Metcalfe 2005). These theories are now valued, particularly during COVID-19 context, due to their ethical nature, their focus on teamwork and partnership and the evidence linked to improved patient care as well as positively enhancing the working environment.

Case Study

Margot disclosed that she wanted to hand in her resignation. As a PNA, I hadn't picked up the discontent before and offered the opportunity for a longer conversation in a quiet space. Margot explained that a new digital medication administration tool had been implemented on the ward, and she had missed some of the training but felt unable to state simply she didn't understand. She thought she was too old to learn new things. I had no idea this had happened and explained that training was still available, and we agreed on an approach forward with structured training and supervision over the next few weeks. I assured her that people learn in different ways and at different paces. We caught up a month later, and Margot had been using the system independently; in fact, she had even shared some shortcut tips with other members of the team and happily settled back into the team.

E-leadership concerns the situation found in more recent situations, where communication is often not on a face-to-face basis, often across various specialties in Trusts across the country and with staff requiring more 'agile working arrangements', especially post-COVID. This results in greater e-communication and thus further challenges for leaders. Building trust, maintaining open lines of communication and being open to subtle cues of concern are crucial in what are seen as virtual working environments. The greater use of Teams/Zoom meetings across various sectors of health services and universities is now evident. Avolio and Kahai (2002) noted in their research that virtual teams may be geographically and culturally spread out. Thus, e-leaders should promote interdependence and reliance to give virtual teams a reason to work successfully together. This leads to the notion of working across various health industry systems.

Systems leadership also concerns collaborative working but across a number of organisational structures to bring about effective improvement. Collective leadership involves taking responsibility for the success of systems in the healthcare organisations involved, with a focus on learning and improving the quality of care delivered to patients and service users (The King's Fund 2015). Macdonald et al. (2016, p. 12) note, however, that systems leadership is also about a social process, so it is more about relationships than power. The 'Magnet' status of excellence reflects how global and international influence can drive patient quality upwards (Jones 2017). Global leadership therefore assists in growing our excellence in care through people empowerment. Manley and Titchen (2017) utilised emancipatory action research with nurses, midwives, health visitors and allied health practitioners who were working at a higher level of practice and recommended that policy makers, governments and commissioners recognise the role of facilitation skills for clinical systems leadership to achieve quality, productivity and effective person-centred services. Scott and Jordon (2023) supported these leadership ideas and related the importance of nurturing staff to drive out negative behaviours that are a consequence of issues that affect staff personally.

CONCLUSION

In conclusion, this chapter has offered a wide range of leadership perspectives that have crossed boundaries with management theories and attempted to apply them to the contemporary PNA role. Transforming and improving services means building up exemplary professional practice through staff support and empowering individuals at all levels to grow in resilience and learn new strategies to deal with complex and demanding work and life challenges.

TIPS FOR PNA PRACTICE

Tip 1: Get the support of your manager and ensure you get protected time to undertake your role. This is the key reason why PNA role is not embedded.

Tip 2: Promote your role and its benefits to everyone, attend staff meetings and trust network forums to 'sell' the role; otherwise, people will quickly forget it, and the role will suddenly be forgotten. Celebrate success and showcase achievements to stakeholders. Lead by example and show integrity, kindness and a strong work ethic.

Tip 3: Remember you are human, so know your own limitations and the boundaries of the PNA role – how the role fits in with other wellbeing roles within your own speciality. Find or set up your support circle. Networks allow you to reach beyond your service and form connections. Don't forget to look back and reflect on what you are achieving as a PNA – use a reflective diary, share best practice or collaborate with other PNAs.

Tip 4: Listen – This builds trust and is valuable and powerful, which enables staff to share concerns or experiences in a psychologically safe space, building trust, confidence and competence. There is evidence how bottling up emotions contributes to blame, anxiety, guilt and in the long-term burnout.

Tip 5: Build relationships and create a culture where staff feel safe to ask questions and are essential in healthcare; it not only supports individual growth and confidence but also strengthens team performance, prevents errors and fosters a psychologically safe environment where learning, reflection and patient safety thrive. Asking questions helps currency and safety. When one person speaks up, it gives others permission to do the same as others may be wondering the same thing but be too shy to ask. As a questioning leader, this demonstrates vulnerability and integrity and helps create a culture of *psychological safety* where reflection, honesty, and collaboration thrive. Get to know the people around you – HCAs, nurses, admin staff and cleaners. Being approachable and respectful goes a long way. You will find your team more willing to support you if they know you genuinely value them. We know from research around incivility that how we are treated impacts and how we treat the next person – so this stuff is infectious. Start with small conversations, smile, say hello, learn peoples' names, ask how people's days are going and these casual interactions grow over time. Show appreciation, thank colleagues for little things, restocking, helping with tasks.

Tip 6: Look after yourself, make sure you have regular supervision by a professional who is trained to do this. Be a role model of good practice when it comes to your own wellbeing, i.e. don't do RCS in your own time or leave. Your downtime is important too.

Tip 7: Remember your CPD is important, so keep up to date with quality improvement (QI) knowledge and research, such as exploring the evaluation research by Lees-Deutsch et al. 2025.

ACKNOWLEDGEMENT

Many thanks to Heather Price, Amy Kelse, Karen Wilson and Adele Parsons who provided real-life case studies and tips for PNA practice.

REFERENCES

Adair, J. (2010). *Develop Your Leadership Skills*. London: Kogan Page.

Alimo-Metcalfe, B. and Alban-Metcalfe, J. (2005). Leadership: time for a new direction. *Leadership* 1 (1): 51–71.

Avolio, B.J. and Gardner, W.L. (2005). Authentic leadership development: getting to the root of positive forms of leadership. *The Leadership Quarterly* 16: 315–338. https://doi.org/10.1016/j.leaqua.2005.03.001.

Avolio, B.J. and Kahai, S.S. (2002). Adding the "e" to e-leadership: how it may impact your leadership. *Organizational Dynamica* 31 (4): 325–338. https://doi.org/10.1016/S0090-2616(02)00133-X.

Baldwin, B., Coyne, T., and Kelly, P. (2022). Supporting nursing, midwifery and allied health professional teams through restorative clinical supervision. *British Journal of Nursing* 31 (20): 1058–1011.

Barr and Dowding (2026). *Leadership in Health Care*, 6e. London: Sage Publications.

Bass, B. (1985). *Leadership and Performance Beyond Expectations*. New York: Free Press.

Bass, B. and Avolio, B.J. (1990). Developing transformational leadership: 1992 and beyond. *Journal of European Industrial Training* 14: 21–27.

Bennis, W.G. (1999). The leadership advantage. *Leader to Leader* 12 (2): 18–23.

Bennis, W.G., Parikh, J., and Leesom, R. (1994). *Beyond Leadership: Balancing Economics, Ethics and Ecology*. London: Blackwell.

Burns, J.M. (1978). *Leadership*. New York: Harper & Row.

Burns, J.M. (2010). *Leadership*. New York: Harper Perennial Modern Classics.

Covey, S. (2004). *The Seven Habits of Highly Effective People: Powerful Lessons in Personal Change* (15th anniversary edn). London: Simon & Schuster.

Daft, R.L. (2017). *The Leadership Experience*, 6e. Delhi: Cengage.

DoH (1993). *Changing Childbirth: Report of the Expert Maternity Group Pt.1*. London: Stationery Office Books.

Dickinson, H., Snelling, I., Ham, C., and Spurgeon, P. (2017). Are we nearly there yet? *A study of the English National Health Service as professional bureaucracies Journal of Health Organization and Management* 31 (4): 430–444.

Fayol, H. (1925). *General and Industrial Management*. London: Pitman and Sons.

Fiedler, F.E. (1967). *A Theory of Leadership Effectiveness*. New York: McGraw Hill.

Fox, J. (1998). *Employee Empowerment: An Apprenticeship Model*. University of Hartford USA.

George, B. (2003). *Authentic Leadership: Rediscovering the Secrets to Creating Lasting Value*. San Francisco, CA: Jossey-Bass.

Handy, C.B. (1985). *Understanding Organisations*, 3e. Oxford: Oxford University Press.

Harris, J. and Mayo, P. (2018). Taking a case study approach to assessing alternative leadership models in health care. *British Journal of Nursing* 27 (11): 608–613.

Henshaw, A., Clarke, D., and Long, A. (2013). Midwives and supervisors of midwives' perceptions of the statutory supervision of midwifery within the United Kingdom: a systematic review. *Midwifery* 29: 75–85.

Huston, C.J. (2024). *Leadership Roles and Management Functions in Nursing: Theory and Application*, 11e. Philadelphia: Wolters Kluwer.

Johnson, G. and Scholes, K. (1989). *Exploring Corporate Strategy*. London: Prentice Hall.

Jones, K. (2017). The benefits of magnet status for nurses, patients and organisations. *Nursing Times [online]* 113 (11): 28–31.

Kanter, R.M. (1983). *The Change Masters*. London: George Allen.

Kouzes, J. M. and Posner, B. Z. (2007) *The Leadership challenge* (4th Edition) San Francisco, CA: Jossey Bass

Krebs, J.P., Madigan, E.A., and Tullai-McGuinness. (2008). The rural nurse work environment and structural empowerment. *Policy, Politics and Nursing Practice* https://doi.org/10.1177/1527154408316255.

Laschinger, H.K.S. (2010). Towards a comprehensive theory of nurse/patient empowerment applying Kanter's empowerment theory to patient care. *Journal of Nursing Management* 18 (1): 4–13.

Lees-Deutsch, L., Palmer, S., Adegboye, A. et al. (2023). Professional nurse advocates: a national evaluation survey of the programme in England. *BioMed Central Nursing* https://doi.org/10.1186/s12912-025-03415-z.

Lees-Deutsch, L., Kneafsey, R., Palmer, S., and Wilde, L. (2025). *SUStAIN-ING: SUpervision, Support & Advocacy for Improvement in Nursing: A Study to Understand the Impact that PNAs Have on Patient Outcomes and Patient Experience, through Quality Improvement Projects they Lead*. Coventry University ISBN: 978-1-84600-132 1 https://doi.org/10.18552/CHC/2025/0005.

Lewin, K. (1951). *Field Theory in Social Sciences*. New York: Harper & Row.

Macdonald, I., Burke, C., and Stewart, K. (2016). *Systems Leadership: Creating Positive Organisations*. Abingdon: Routledge.

Malby, R. (1994). *The Challenges for Nursing and Midwifery in the 21st Century: A Briefing Document*. Leeds: University of Leeds.

Manley, K. and Titchen, A. (2017). Facilitation skills: the catalyst for increased effectiveness in consultant practice and clinical systems leadership. *Educational Action Research* 25 (2): 256–279.

Mintzberg, H. (1998). 5 Ps for strategy. In: *The Strategy Process* (rev. European edn) (ed. H. Mintzberg, J. Quinn, and S. Ghoshal). Englewood Cliffs, NJ: Prentice Hall.

Mubarak, F. and Noor, A. (2018). Effect of authentic leadership on employee creativity in project-based organizations with the mediating roles of work engagement and psychological empowerment. *Cogent Business and Management* 5 (1).

Northouse, P.G. (2016). *Leadership: Theory and Practice*, 7e. London: Sage.

Nursing and Midwifery Council (NMC) (2018a). *The Code: Professional Standards of Practice and Behaviour for Nurses, Midwives and Nursing Associates*. London: NMC.

Nursing and Midwifery Council (NMC) (2018b). *Realising Professionalism: Standards for Education and Training, Part 3: Standards for Pre-Registration Programmes*. London: NMC.

Nursing and Midwifery Council (NMC) (2018c). *Realising Professionalism: Standards for Education and Training – Standards for Pre-Registration Nursing Associates Programmes*. London: NMC.

Nursing and Midwifery Council (NMC) (2018d). *Standards of Proficiency for Registered Nurses*. London: NMC.

Royal College of Nursing (RCN) (2023). *Professional Nurse Advocate Standards for Education and Training Programmes and Modules*. London: RCN.

Schein, E.H. (1985). *Organizational Culture and Leadership*. San Francisco, CA: Jossey-Bass.

Schein, E.H. (1992). Coming to a new awareness of organizational culture. In: *Human Resource Strategies* (ed. G. Salaman). London: Sage.

Scott, I. (1998). Challenging the future. *Nursing Management* 4 (9): 18–21.

Scott, A. and Jordon, S. (2023). Leadership and management in healthcare: using theory to motivate staff to achieve organisational goals. *International Journal of Advancing Practice* 1 (1): 33–36.

Short R chairman (1980). *Perinatal and Neonatal Mortality. Second Report from the Social Services Committee 1979–80.* London: HMSO.

Tannenbaum, R. and Schmidt, W.H. (1958). How to choose a leadership pattern. *Harvard Business Review* 36: 95–101.

The King's Fund (2015). The practice of system leadership: being comfortable with chaos. www.kingsfund.org.uk/insight-and-analysis/reports/practice-system-leadership (accessed 13 June 2025).

Vroom, V.H. and Jago, A.G. (1988). *The New Leadership.* Englewood Cliffs, NJ: Prentice Hall.

Wagner, A., Pollack, P., and Swiatkiewicz-Mosny, M. (2019). Who defines – who decides? Theorising the epistemic communities, communities of practice and interest groups in the healthcare field: a discursive approach. *Social Theory and Health Journal* 17: 192–212.

Walker, W., Smythe, A., Lees-Deutsch, L. et al. (2025). The personal and professional impacts of becoming and being a professional nurse advocate. *British Journal of Nursing* 34 (6): 336–344. https://doi.org/10.12968/bjon.2024.0249.

Wallbank, S. and Woods, G. (2012). A healthier health visiting workforce: findings from the restorative clinical supervision programme. *Community Practitioner* 85 (11): 20–23.

Wallbank, S. and Woods, G. (2013). Reflecting on leadership in health visiting and the restorative model of supervision. *Journal of Health Visiting* 1 (3): 173–176. http://Magonlinelibrary.com.

Weber, M. (1921). *Economy and Society: An Outline of Interpretive Sociology,* vol. 2 Vols. Berkeley, CA: University of California Press.

Weitz, R., Brinkerhoft, D., White, L.K., and Ortega, S.T. (2011). *Essentials of Sociology,* 9e. Boston, MA: Cengage Learning India Pvt Ltd.

West, M.A. (2024). *Compassionate Leadership: Sustaining Wisdom, Humanity and Presence in Health and Social Care.* London: The Swirling Leaf Press.

White, R.K. and Lippitt, R. (2006[1960])Autocracy and democracy: an experimental inquiry. In: *Leadership Roles and Management Functions in Nursing: Theory and Application,* 5e (ed. B.L. Marquis and C.J. Huston). Philadelphia, PA: Lippincott.

Williams, E. and Hunt, S. (1996). Supervision in midwifery practice: the debate and some evidence. *British Journal of Midwifery* 4 (1): 28–31.

CHAPTER 4

A-EQUIP – Exploring the Normative Aspects of the Model (Education and Development)

Clare Capito

NHS England, London, UK

A-EQUIP MODEL EDUCATION AND DEVELOPMENT

The purpose of this chapter is to provide an overview of the A-EQUIP model of supervision and the attributes and development required for a professional nurse advocate (PNA) to be able to deploy the model. There will be several case studies throughout this chapter that will illustrate how PNAs have implemented the A-EQUIP model, as well as case studies that demonstrate how a function of the model has been utilised.

The A-EQUIP model is made up of four distinct functions: normative, restorative, personal action for quality improvement and education, and development; see Figure 4.1 (Flack and Abdulmohdi 2023). All four functions have equal importance and value and can be used together or independently.

It was originally designed in 2017 by NHS England (NHSE) as a new model of midwifery supervision to replace statutory supervision as described in Chapter 2. It is anticipated that through the use of the A-EQUIP model of clinical supervision, staff will feel empowered and developed, as well as the quality of care they provide will improve and that this will

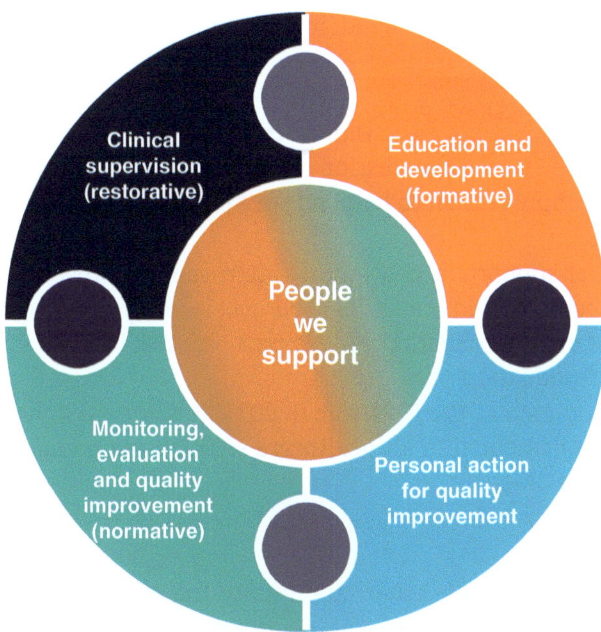

FIGURE 4.1 A-EQUIP model infographic. *Source:* Adapted by Flack and Abdulmohdi (2023) from NHS England (2017).

promote the A-EQUIP model as 'an intrinsic part of everyone's job, every day in all parts of the system' (NHS England 2017).

The A-EQUIP model stems from Proctor's model of clinical supervision (1987), which has been used in health services:

- **Normative Function of Monitoring, Evaluation and Quality Control:** this applies to managerial aspects concerning practice, learning and core mandatory training
- **Formative Function of Education and Development:** this applies to the educational aspects, reviewing how the practitioner develops their knowledge and skills and self-reflection, as well as considering their nursing career and progression
- **Restorative Function of Restorative Clinical Supervision:** this applies to supportive aspects, which include personal development, improving stress management and mitigating burnout.

A fourth function was added in 2017 with the development of the A-EQUIP model:

- **Personal Action for Quality Improvement:** this addresses the need for healthcare professional to be familiar with and contribute to quality improvement to help improve patient care.

The model supports a continuous improvement process that aims to build on the personal and professional clinical leadership of nurses, enhance the quality of care for patients, and support preparedness for appraisal and professional revalidation.

Since the launch of the PNA role in 2021, it is apparent that a PNA service can be implemented in all healthcare settings, including the following fields of nursing practice:

- Critical care
- Children's nursing – acute, community and mental health
- Mental health – both acute and in the community
- Acute nursing, including palliative care
- Community nursing – including health visiting, district nursing and school nursing
- Learning disability
- Health in the justice system

The A-EQUIP model is flexible and can be implemented according to organisational requirements to support collaboration between nurses and healthcare colleagues when delivering restorative clinical supervision (RCS) sessions. Support for implementation of a PNA service is obtained by the NHS Standard Contract 2025/2026 (NHS England 2024), which states that each Trust should have professional leadership that is appropriate to the service in relation to clinical supervision for nurses that is aligned to the A-EQUIP model.

Furthermore, the NHS People Plan (2020/2021) and NHS England's Long Term Workforce Plan (NHS England 2023) recommend that 'focussed support for staff wellbeing through restorative supervision has a positive impact' on staff, as well as the patients and people that they support. The following case study from Oxleas NHS Foundation Trust illustrates how a PNA service can be successfully implemented across several health care settings in several locations.

Oxleas' PNA Journey: How Does the PNA Service Remain Visible Across 125 Sites Spread Across the Southeast and Southwest of England?

Oxleas is a diverse NHS Foundation Trust with nurses in adults' and children's mental and physical health, learning disabilities, forensics and offender health care. There are approximately 1400 nurses who work across 125 sites. Our geographic footprint spreads from SE London (Greenwich, Bexley and Bromley) to Prison Services in Kent, Devon, Dorset, Bristol and Wiltshire.

Our PNA journey started in 2021, with the launch of our steering group and exploring how we can develop the PNA service as we had put forward many nurses to train as PNAs and our nursing leadership was fully supportive and in 2022, our Associate Director of Nursing at the time contributed to working on the stakeholder group for the development of the Royal College of Nursing (RCN) PNA training standards.

The real 'PNA Explosion', as we call it, was when we carried out a large marketing campaign highlighting the A-EQUIP focus of our PNA workforce, showcasing the PNA's focus on advocacy and improvement of the experience of being a nurse in Oxleas. This was done by carrying out trust-wide listening lounges; our listening lounges were an idea from one of our first cohort of PNAs, and the idea was to visit clinical areas and have a drop-in clinic in the afternoon; we spent the morning visiting staff, helping where we could and explaining the PNA role, and then listening to their concerns or issues in the afternoon.

Along with our listening lounges, we created a video explaining the PNA role and owning our strapline, 'Nurses looking after nurses'. In our video, we had nurses from our chief nurse, Jane, to junior staff nurses explaining the PNA role and how it can improve their experience in Oxleas with a focus on the skills in restorative clinical supervision and career conversations.

Following on from our 'PNA Explosion', the PNA service in Oxleas has gone from strength to strength; we work closely with human resources to ensure that staff trust-wide have access to an offer of support from a PNA. Furthermore, the Trust has funded 28 PNA training places and

(continued)

(*continued*)

commissioned a university partner to deliver this. Amongst those who will attend this course, is our chief nurse and two heads of nursing, thus making our PNA offer 'From Ward to Board'. Further funding has been identified to upskill 36 of our experienced PNAs with continuing professional development (CPD) opportunities.

As part of our PNA offer, we support on average 49 nurses a month, and in 1 year (Nov 23–Nov 24) we supported 588 nurses, roughly 40% of the nursing workforce!

Our Top Tips for Implementing a PNA Service in Your Trust

- Find your early adopters, take them on the journey, be brave and try ideas that seem outlandish.
- Have a story and a focus, be authentic and own it.
- Get your wellbeing teams involved and showcase to human resources (HR) the benefit of this to the nursing workforce.
- Track your data diligently and use it to reinforce your story.
- Don't have a PNA leader, have a PNA community.

Thank you to every Oxleas' PNA who has assisted our PNA journey!

Jake Chambers, PNA Trust Lead, Oxleas NHS Foundation Trust

THE NORMATIVE FUNCTION OF THE A-EQUIP MODEL: MONITORING, EVALUATION AND QUALITY IMPROVEMENT

This function focuses on the supervisee developing their clinical skills and accountability, so that they become more effective in their clinical role. The PNA role facilitates this by providing the supervisee with opportunities to reflect, discuss a clinical situation or an incident and then for the supervisee to determine what further learning or action may be required.

The benefits of this function include (NHS England 2022):

- Promotes professional accountability.
- Promotes involvement in improving quality issues.
- Improves effectiveness in a clinical role.
- Supports service improvement to deliver a high standard of patient care.

THE FORMATIVE FUNCTION OF THE A-EQUIP MODEL: EDUCATIONAL AND DEVELOPMENT

This function focuses on the development of a supervisee's skills, knowledge, attitudes and self-reflection, which is facilitated by the PNA.

When the PNA facilitates an RCS, the supervisee can undertake self-reflection and explore their own leadership skills and qualities through examining their interactions with others within a situation or issue. This discussion with a PNA in a safe space can encourage the supervisee to influence change and improve the standard of care being delivered.

Thus, reflection on practice is key for a supervisee to develop insights into their strengths and weaknesses and identify areas that require improvement or need to be developed, and this is vital for a supervisee fulfilling their revalidation requirements with the Nursing Midwifery Council (NMC). The NMC Revalidation resources have reflection templates (reflective-accounts-form.doc), which are useful for the supervisee to complete following a discussion and reflection with a PNA and include as part of their revalidation.

There are many reflection models that can be used to assist with a reflective discussion, and one of the most popular appears to be Gibbs Reflective Cycle (Gibbs' Reflective Cycle | Reflection Toolkit) and other models of reflection can be found here: `https://www.google.co.uk/url?sa=t&rct=j&q=&esrc=s&source=web&cd=&ved=2ahUKEwjUgMDpt5OMAxWVSkEAHRRAASwQFnoECAwQAQ&url=https%3A%2F%2Flibguides.cam.ac.uk%2Freflectivepracticetoolkit%2Fmodels&usg=AOvVaw3c2on9FjIzVi2d_U_NFZ7o&opi=89978449`

THE RESTORATIVE FUNCTION OF THE A-EQUIP MODEL: RESTORATIVE CLINICAL SUPERVISION

This function focuses on the well-being of the workforce, providing support and reflection for the supervisee in a psychologically safe environment. For instance, if an 'event' or 'issue' occurs, the supervisee can meet with the PNA for an RCS session, where learning and reflection would be encouraged (Pettit et al. 2015). RCS has been shown to be effective in reducing stress and burnout and increasing compassion satisfaction (Wallbank and Woods 2012) as well as providing a strategy to mitigate workplace stress, which will enhance retention and 'assists with the management of personal and professional demands' (RCN 2021).

There is evidence that staff are coming to work even though they may be ill and therefore not fully functioning while at work and could also be more prone to making errors. This is also known as presenteeism and RCS can support this by exploring the issues that are affecting the supervisee/member of staff and discover what lies behind their presenteeism; thus, active listening is an essential skill for a PNA to possess.

It is important to remember that the PNA needs to signpost the supervisee for further psychological support if there is a great amount of emotional distress being discussed or observed, e.g. suicidal ideation.

The table below outlines the recommended actions that the PNA should undertake according to the severity of the situation.

Recommended PNA Actions for Signposting Support

Support/Signpost

Serious Concerns and supervisee is with the PNA	Contact emergency services on 111 or 999 or the Accident and Emergency department if there is one on-site
Treat as a crisis	
Serious concerns but supervisee is off-site	Is not responding to contact which is unusual for this person?
	Has anyone else in the team been in contact with them? Could you discreetly ask someone who knows them well to reach out?
	If no one in the team is able to reach them, call their next of kin to check that they are ok? Be discreet
	If you are unable to make contact/establish safety
Treat as a crisis	AND have reason to believe they are at risk, call the police on 101 and ask them to conduct a welfare check
Less serious concerns	Provide the number for the local Mental Health Crisis line
	Also, provide the following support lines:
Thoughts only	Samaritans: 24/7 helpline: 116 123
	The Listening Place: Counselling for people with thoughts of suicide 02023 906 7676
	Refer to Occupational Health for a psychological assessment

(Continued)

No thoughts of suicide or self-harm	Signpost to: Staff counselling Text 'SHOUT' to 85258 for a 24/7 response
But expressing mental health difficulties	Refer to Occupational Health for a psychological assessment
Follow-up	
Check-in	Contact the supervisee within 24 hours to ask how they are now, has additional support been offered, is any further escalation required?
Report	Where necessary and appropriate escalate to senior colleagues/teams with the supervisee's permission and knowledge.

The next case study provides an example of RCS session facilitated by a PNA and how it assisted a nurse to reflect and view a challenging situation in a different way which they found beneficial. The PNA reflected upon the insight she gained which enhanced her learning when undertaking an RCS session.

Restorative Clinical Supervision (RCS) with a Member of Team Following an Outburst at a Team Meeting

Nurse A was showing signs of stress and burnout, and it was affecting the working relationships within the unit. As a small nursing team, we have different strengths and worked well together, but Nurse A had become emotional, reserved and had isolated themselves. It is important that every member of the team can maintain professionalism and be given the opportunity to reflect upon the challenges that they may be experiencing.

Therefore, time was allocated for Nurse A to meet with the PNA for an RCS session; this would provide a safe space for them to look at the issues and concerns that they may be experiencing. The PNA does not counsel but instead listens to the supervisee, enabling them to address professional and emotional challenges in new and innovative ways and thus developing a resilient and engaged supervisee.

(continued)

(*continued*)

During the RCS session, Nurse A was able to reflect upon how they were struggling with the dynamics within the team, and this was causing their own stress. However, being listened to, supported and challenged gently by the PNA, Nurse A reflected that this had assisted them and improved their capacity to cope better at work.

PNA's Reflection

Completing this one to one RCS has given me more of an insight into benefits of RCS sessions. In the role of a PNA, we need to ask questions and gently probe around issues, which allows the supervisee the opportunity to see things from a different perspective.

The restorative function of the A-EQUIP model is the lynch pin of the model, and because its implementation is employer-led, there can be a variation in the RCS offer, which leads to variation of its effectiveness and outcome (Capito et al. 2022).

The following table provides how RCS can be arranged:

Restorative Clinical Supervision (RCS) Sessions	
1–1	Provides individual support for the supervisee to reflect and consider a situation and the learning they have obtained.
Group (maximum of eight attendees)	Offers shared reflection and learning. It is often comforting for supervisees to hear from their colleagues and to realise that they are experiencing something similar.
Opportunistic/ Check-in	This can sometimes be easier for team members/ colleagues to speak in the moment, which offers an opportunity for the staff member to be heard and feel valued. As a follow-up, the supervisee may need to book an RCS session to explore an issue in more depth.
Restorative Conversations	Ad hoc conversations with a practitioner, which may require no further action or require a follow-up RCS session.

RCS can be opportunistic and not always booked via a 'clinic', and anecdotally, this appears to be the most common approach to RCS. This correlates with the work by Neil Greenberg on the PIES (P = Proximal, I = immediate, E = expect an end, S = keep it simple) model (Greenberg and Tracy, 2020), which is an evidence-based model to use in practice to build resilience for staff to cope with distress, to de-escalate before it becomes a bigger problem.

Greenburg suggests that being assigned a buddy to monitor each other's well-being can support staff in practice with their emotional well-being. This would fit well with RCS sessions provided by a PNA, as just being there to actively listen or having someone to talk to and bounce ideas off.

Active listening, as part of communication skills, is essential for a leader to possess, enabling them to confidently contact those who are displaying signs of presenteeism. Greenberg and Tracy (2020) discuss in their paper that leaders need to encourage social bonds between colleagues and supervisors or professional advocates, as this is protective of mental health and supports colleagues/staff with signs of presenteeism, which is reported to be a larger problem than absenteeism. As far back as 1959, Herzberg explored in his two-factor theory that job dissatisfaction can be present if motivating factors are not managed well. Herzberg's work appears to agree with the presenteeism noted by Greenberg. Herzberg's work discusses that a lack of job satisfiers doesn't always lead to dissatisfaction and poor performance; it may merely lead to workers doing an adequate job, rather than their best (Presenteeism).

RCS can support with presenteeism and absenteeism in practice, exploring any issues affecting the team member/colleague or, indeed, nursing students, to discover what lies behind the presenteeism or absenteeism. Consideration should be given to the notion that RCS doesn't need to be a booked session; often opportunistic discussions led or guided by the principles of A-EQUIP and RCS are often all that is needed to contain the staff member.

A testimonial shared at the London PNA conference in 2024 by an attendee:

The PNA was very professional in their approach, took time to listen and really understood my concerns. They skilfully guided the conversation to ensure all my concerns were addressed. We also discussed career opportunities and there was time to look through current job roles advertised within the trust that might suit my preferences-this exceeded my expectations.

The following case study provides the results of an audit of nurses who were new to working in the Oncology department who had been provided with RCS sessions with a PNA and how they valued this.

Background

This case study aims to introduce clinical supervision as a 'safe space' for nurses on the oncology ward by a professional nurse advocate.

Aim

To provide restorative clinical supervision (RCS) sessions to nurses working in the Oncology department to address and reduce any compassion fatigue. RCS contains elements of psychological support, including listening, supporting, and challenging the supervisee to improve their capacity to cope, especially in managing difficult and stressful situations.

Method

- RCS sessions were commenced for all new nurses in the Oncology department from December 2022, and a 'safe space' was created.
- Trained PNAs provided the RCS sessions, and they were provided either to individual nurses or in closed groups comprising two to three nurses.
- The RCS session was provided online via MS Teams or face to face.
- The PNAs met with the nurses once a month for a 1-hour period for 6 months. This 1 hour was allocated in the nurse's rota to ensure their availability and attendance.
- The PNA provided anonymised feedback to the senior management team about the themes that were discussed. In addition, the PNAs provided resources and support for the nurses, including referrals to occupational health.
- The PNA also supported the nurses with any quality improvement works that may have been discussed in the clinical supervision session.
- The Clinical Supervision Evaluation Questionnaire (CSEQ) was used to measure the effectiveness of the clinical supervision.

Implementation

The RCS sessions ran for a total of 18 formal group sessions over 6 months.

The effectiveness of restorative clinical supervision was measured by CSEQ. Scoring was as follows:

- Above 14 indicates a strong positive perception of the RCS session as a group.

- Score above 0 indicates a positive perception.
- A score below 0 shows that the attendees had a negative perception of the RCS session.

Results of CESQ

All the scores were above 0, which indicates all the respondents had a positive perception of restorative clinical supervision.

The staff members also provided very positive feedback and wanted to attend more sessions in the future.

Actions Taken From the Sessions Over the 6 Months

✓ Three nurses needed further emotional support and were signposted to University College London Hospital (UCLH) SPAWS (staff psychologic and well-being services), and one staff member had a GP appointment.

✓ One nurse needed financial support and was signposted to different charities and the UCLH staff experience team.

✓ One nurse started participating in the quality improvement (QI) project in the ward.

✓ One nurse was offered support for revalidation.

✓ Two career conversations took place.

✓ Three nurses had further education and training needs identified, and therefore, training was put in place for them.

Implications

This audit demonstrated that the professional nurse advocate role was key in supporting these nurses new to working in the Oncology department, assisted in improving their personal and professional development and had a direct effect on their well-being, thus improving patient experience.

Dominic Maprany Devassy, PNA, Oncology Department, University College London Hospital

PERSONAL ACTION FOR QUALITY IMPROVEMENT FUNCTION OF THE A-EQUIP MODEL

To improve patient care, it is important that nurses become familiar with and contribute to quality improvement, as this is a fundamental aspect of the nurse's role.

This function 'ensures that the improvement of quality care becomes part of everyone's role, every day, across the system' (NHS 2017).

Benefits for nurses' personal contribution to quality improvement may include:

- Opportunities where the nurse has reflected, learned and taught others about their personal action for QI
- Participation in audit and research, and contribution to the implementation of findings where appropriate
- Embedding learning from incidents
- Contributing to service improvements because of feedback from patients and/or staff

Lees-Deutsch et al. (2025), in their research SUSTAIN-ING, explore the many ways in which QI has been introduced into the work of the PNA.

Launching and Implementing Professional Advocacy Service in Princess Alexandra Hospital Trust

Silpa Dhaneesh, PNA Trust Lead

In 2020, the results of the staff survey at Princess Alexandra Hospital Trust (PAHT) reported a significant decline in staff engagement and morale, which was attributed to the unprecedented pressures faced by nursing staff during the COVID-19 pandemic.

Launching the Professional Nurse Advocacy Service Initiative Involved the Following Stakeholders

- Professional nurse advocates (PNAs)
- Health and Well-being team
- Freedom to Speak Up Guardians
- Library services
- 'Here for You' initiative
- Nursing staff within the organisation

Silpa assumed her role as the Trust PNA lead in August 2022 with the goal of unifying professional nurse advocates working in the Trust under a structured framework aimed at promoting education and implementing the A-EQUIP model of supervision. Therefore, Silpa arranged the following activities to promote and strengthen the PNA role and PNA service at PAHT:

1. Engaged in one-on-one discussions with PNAs to clarify roles and responsibilities.
2. Developed a PNA contract allocating 7.5 hours per month to each PNA.
3. Launched a 'Trolley Dash' campaign for increased service visibility and awareness.
4. Introduced keychains with quick response (QR) codes for immediate access to team resources.
5. Established a network with various stakeholders.
6. Organised Career Clinics to support professional growth discussions.
7. Initiated Well-being Weeks to enhance awareness of well-being services and create safe spaces for dialogue.
8. Scheduled away days for team well-being promotion.
9. Implemented a transparent recruitment process for PNA students and created a dedicated student hub.
10. Established a buddy system for clinical supervision among PNAs.
11. Formed a steering group for PNAs.
12. Conducted a full-day Career Workshop and developed a career workbook for nurses.
13. Launched 90-day preceptorships for PNAs.
14. Initiated monthly newsletters for staff updates.
15. Developed a professional advocacy strategy for 2024–2026.
16. Developed SOP for providing restorative clinical supervision.
17. Expanded advocacy efforts to include Allied Health Professionals (AHPs).
18. Provided in-house training on quality improvement fundamentals for PNAs.

(*continued*)

(*continued*)

In 2023, Staff Were Surveyed, and Staff Morale and Engagement have Improved Since 2021 and Demonstrated That

✓ Significant improvement in staff morale and engagement levels in the follow-up survey.

✓ Positive feedback regarding well-being initiatives from staff.

✓ Enhancement in professional resilience, career development, and quality improvement across the organisation as indicated by qualitative feedback.

✓ 90% of staff believed the PNA service could positively influence retention, with 98% feeling valued and appreciated.

✓ Empowerment among internationally recruited nurses.

✓ Improved professional development across the organisation.

The PAHT 2030 vision is about transforming the way in which healthcare is delivered for our communities and creating a much more modern, much more welcoming place for our patients to be treated and our people to work. It is evident that staff well-being directly affects retention and reduces sickness, which has an impact on patient experience.

Quality Improvement Tools Used to Assist in This Change

✓ Kotter's eight stage change management model was used to launch and implement the service.

✓ Plan do study act (PDSA) cycle and SWOT (Strengths, Weaknesses, Opportunities, and Threats) analysis were done during each stage.

✓ John Fisher's transitional curve to analyse and support staff behaviour throughout the change management.

Key Learning Points for Silpa

• Staff feedback is essential and needs to be acknowledged always.

• Internal network and stakeholder involvement are essential.

• Communication and buy-in from the senior leadership team (SLT).

• Any well-being initiative should be based on identified gaps and in relation to the Trust Vision.

• Stakeholder support and internal/external network are significant in the implementation and sustainability of the service.

THE QUALITIES REQUIRED BY A PNA TO DEPLOY THE A-EQUIP MODEL

Principally, the PNA role guides and supports nurses by deploying the A-EQUIP model, where all four functions have equal importance and value and can be used together or independently. The essential attributes that are required of a PNA consist of integrity, openness, and being able to actively listen, as is upholding the professional standards of practice and behaviour within the Nursing and Midwifery Code (NMC 2018).

The PNA training programme provides nurses with the skills, competencies and confidence to lead programmes of improvement, fostering a culture of learning and development within their clinical settings, and to deliver RCS to their colleagues. The Royal College of Nursing and stakeholders have developed education standards for PNA training (RCN 2023) to provide consistency and reduce variation for Higher Education Institutes to deliver a PNA training programme.

NHS England (2023) has specified application criteria for nurses to train as a PNA, which has been in the main funded by NHS England, but the features for PNA training are the following:

- Professional development at master's level 7 with a national qualification in leadership and advocacy
- Each student PNA will have access to a supervisor (qualified PNA) provided by their employing organisation
- Curriculum for PNA training is based upon the RCN standards (2023)
- Virtual classes over a 10-week period to measure competency using chosen forms of assessment

As part of the Professional Nursing Advocate module, I completed a presentation on active listening. A concept was born for the implementation of Restorative Clinical Supervision (RCS) within the Ambulance

(continued)

(continued)

Service called the 'In the Cab' (ITC) model. This delivers restorative clinical conversations in the:

- cab
- car
- classroom
- control room

RCS is one element of the A-EQUIP model (Advocating & Educating for Quality Improvement) and is for all areas of our Ambulance workforce and for all grades of staff.

The rationale behind this approach was how, as an ambulance service which is predominantly mobile, remote & under constant extreme pressure could increase opportunities for listening and reflection to staff/volunteers. The benefits of this are that it can improve morale & enable staff to speak up about things that may be impacting their delivery of patient care. We know that releasing staff from duties is a difficult task with the current operational pressures the NHS is facing. However, if we do not look after staff, we cannot care for patients.

My idea was that an RCS conversation could take place within the shift rather than adopting a set time and place for staff to attend. This made the model more attractive and able to meet ambulance operational models.

The second model of delivery of Restorative clinical supervision is being used within our Ambulance Emergency Operations Centre (EOC), which are our emergency control rooms that receive 999 calls and dispatch ambulances. The model works on the use of set time slots offered for staff to book onto. This model works better within the control room as the staff are within one space for a period of time and cover can be provided by other staff.

A Q & A sheet is given to all members of staff/volunteers prior to the session, which will give guidance of what the session will involve. These include a confidentiality statement, what to expect during the session & the three anonymous questions that will be asked.

1. What two things can improve for your experience at work?
2. What are you most proud of this month?
3. What has been challenging saying yes to?

Following the session, a pack is handed out with signposting information for staff to refer to in their own time if needed. I have also included a positive affirmation card for each pack.

This model has been included in our Clinical Supervision policy & themes & trends reported to our Board.

All PNA training programmes are taught via online platforms, and therefore the content must be meaningful to the student PNA and encourage them to be motivated to complete the assigned learning. Consideration also needs to be given to the fact that adult learners may have different learning styles and learning needs, including neurodiversity; hence, a variety of teaching techniques should be employed to ensure that the teaching methods are inclusive of all learning needs or preferences.

Case Study: PNA Training Programme at Anglia Ruskin University (ARU)

We offer a 10-week, master's level (level 7) online module to prepare participants/students for the PNA role in practice, supported by the theory. We have trained over 2000 PNAs though our module. Although online learning does not suit everyone, active learning is included which assists in improving understanding and information retention (Konopka et al. 2015 cited work from).

We strive to offer active learning by using interactive tools within sessions. Furthermore, we have found it to be beneficial to teach Midwives, Midwives from the Higher Midwifery Pathway, Nurses, Allied health professionals (AHP) and apprentices from our advanced clinical practice pathway for apprentices (ACP) together as this provides rich discussions and allows for peer learning to take place.

At ARU, we are aware that some students are often 'sent' or 'chosen' to attend the module; therefore, the module needs to ensure the students have a good understanding of the PNA role and the benefits of RCS. Increasing their understanding of the role and the A-EQUIP model will support them to be motivated to increase their appetite to learn, including considering topics from another perspective and how this will shape what support they can offer in practice to support staff/colleagues through RCS.

Students' thoughts and ideas are pivotal when designing presentations for the module to ensure it meets all their learning needs. Peer learning is evident through the discussions we facilitate on the module at ARU, as students are taught together, they can share with others in the group appropriate examples or just tips from their vast experiences for all to learn from. The learning is designed to support the students to explore new approaches, learning from differing perspectives, and are designed to be thought-provoking, encouraging students to extend and increase their knowledge/learning for the PNA role in practice.

We have key speakers, who are experienced and have a passion for the topic delivered each week; these sessions are like building blocks which increase the students' knowledge and skills, which in turn will increase their confidence to deliver the RCS sessions. Each week, students will view each topic from a different perspective, which encourages reflection and the appetite to learn more about the topic to deepen learning. Student feedback is used to inform future modules and is generally positive.

We often have students who have completed the module, requesting to return to share their experiences in practice which bolsters the current students' understanding of what can be achieved in the PNA role in practice. For instance, they have shared that opportunistic reflective discussions with staff are often better than providing an appointment for a future date. This supports Greenberg and Tracy's (2020) work on the PIES model, which encourages staff close to the frontline to ask for and receive support at the time when they need it.

Session delivery by someone who has experienced the challenges that can be faced when embedding the PNA role into practice makes it more realistic for the students.

Linda Flack, Senior Lecturer in adult nursing, Anglia Ruskin University

The PNA training programmes focus on the leadership skills that are required of a PNA, where they have an opportunity to reflect upon their personal self-awareness and open-mindedness and to understand their own emotions alongside recognising and influencing those emotions within others. Acquiring this knowledge assists PNAs to develop their skills as a compassionate leader and thus create a platform of psychological safety, which in turn promotes an optimal workplace culture for individuals to learn, develop and perform at their best (Kings Fund 2020).

It is vital for the PNA to create a safe and effective space for supervisees who are likely to be experiencing burnout, compassion fatigue, moral distress or moral injury – for more information, please see the text box.

Moral Distress

Psychological Discomfort that Occurs

- when a professional is unable to deliver care in the way that feels ethically correct
- or they are in a situation or moral uncertainty/facing an ethical dilemma.

Moral Injury

Results from prolonged moral distress involve impaired functioning and psychological difficulties.

Core Moral Injury Symptoms in Nurses Include

- guilt (67%),
- shame (71%) and
- loss of trust (50%).

Secondary Symptoms Include

- depression (33%),
- anxiety (57%),
- self-harm (19%),
- anger (71%),
- spiritual-existential crisis (9%),
- social problems (48%).

(Stovall et al. 2020).

Moral Injury & Distress are not considered to be mental illnesses, but the symptoms are often a precursor to post-traumatic stress disorder **(PTSD).**

The Foundation of Nursing Studies (FONS) has developed Resilience-Based Clinical Supervision (RBCS), and this approach to supervision and support aligns closely with RCS and is complementary to the PNA role. RBCS is based upon the principles of compassion-focussed therapy (FONS 23), which acknowledges that all our behaviours are motivated by three emotional systems (see the box below) as identified by Gilbert (2010) and they are guided by 'a desire to compete with the self or others for external validation and success, to soothe the self to enable contentment and self-acceptance, and to protect the self from threat'.

Many PNAs have undertaken additional training in RBCS and utilise the methods they recommend, which acknowledge the emotional systems and how to 'bring the supervisee into the room', particularly if they are very stressed by creating the conditions and framework that allows a supervisee to engage in the RCS session.

The Five Stages of RBCS Are
1. To create a safe space agreement
2. Undertake a grounding exercise, e.g. mindfulness
3. To check-in
4. To have a reflective discussion
5. To spend the last 5–10 minutes of the session for the supervisee to reflect upon the session and any action they will undertake – known as the ending

Three Emotional Regulation Systems

Threat System: the most powerful system, it' primitive, protective and instinctive. It seeks to protect us from physical and social threats – fight, flight, freeze or appease.

Drive System: This is our incentivised system, it is resource focussed and can be what 'gets us up' in the morning. If it goes into overdrive, it can lead to stress, perfectionism and burnout.

Affiliated System: or soothing system, linked to that peaceful, contented state of well-being, we feel connected to others. It's related to giving and receiving care and kindness and love. It allows us to soothe ourselves and others.

FONS (2023)

Compassionate leadership provided by the PNA inevitably requires them to consider their own self-care, as there is often psychological wear and tear (Smith 2021) and this has been acknowledged by NHS England, funding a programme of continuous professional development for PNAs. Also, each region in England hosts either support networks or communities of practice for PNAs to network with other PNAs, sharing the successes and challenges of implementing the PNA role.

It has also become apparent that newly qualified PNAs require programmes of support and mentorship, and the case study below demonstrates an initiative that has been introduced into the Princess Alexandra Hospital Trust to support their newly qualified PNAs.

This Case Study Provides How a PNA Trust Lead has Developed a Resource to Support Newly Qualified PNA

A Booklet to Guide for Newly Qualified Professional Nurse Advocates

Following discussions with student PNAs and those who are newly qualified, it became apparent that there was a gap in coaching and mentorship for newly recruited PNAs.

In response, I have developed this guide, which includes valuable information, resources, and a 90-day checklist designed to support a PNA during their first 3 to 6 months post qualification.

As PNAs embark on their journey, it is essential to recognise that competence, confidence, and passion are the cornerstone attributes that will empower them to become effective role models and advocates. Their role in professional advocacy is not only crucial for our organisation but also holds the potential to significantly enhance both staff well-being and retention, as well as the quality of care we provide to our patients.

This guide is thoughtfully crafted to offer a robust foundation, and it encourages them to engage with mentors and colleagues, fostering a culture of shared experiences and support. Restorative clinical supervision will play a vital role in their own professional development, offering opportunities to reflect on their practice and gain constructive feedback.

The guide was distributed among the professional nurse advocates, undergoing a thorough peer review and receiving approval from the steering group prior to distribution. Each PNA has been provided with a copy, and newly qualified PNAs have been actively utilising the guide since

(continued)

(*continued*)

October 2024. The draft of the booklet has been sent to the communications team for development in the Trust-approved format. Once finalised, this resource will be implemented organisation-wide for PNA, PMA, and PAHPA. This guide is used for Professional Nurse Advocates, Professional Midwifery advocates and Professional AHP advocates and can be adapted easily for all three workforces

The Feedback Received So Far

✓ I have benefited from having the guide since newly qualifying in September as a PNA as it gives you timelines to work to complete the initial steps and gives you a foundation at which to start. I think without it I would have felt quite lost at what to do next. I am a person that likes lists too!

✓ Putting in pictures of the PNAs in the Trust is a good way of identifying them for me, especially as I don't remember names very well.

✓ When newly qualified, an RCS can seem daunting so being able to shadow other PNAs and having the RCS guide provided as well as all the other reflective examples, will all help to give me more direction.

✓ A very informative and useful PA resource. Thank you.

Silpa Dhaneesh, PNA Trust Lead

This chapter has focussed upon the implementation of the A-EQUIP model, and how it can support nurses, healthcare organisations and patients. Each of the four functions has been discussed, which has demonstrated its adaptability and principles linking to national policy. All four functions have equal importance and value and can be used together or independently.

With the use of case studies, it is possible there is information on how a PNA continues with their professional development and how this links to skills, knowledge and experiences to identify self-leadership and the positive impact on self, others and the standard of care provided.

REFERENCES

Capito, C., Keegan, C., Lachanudis, L. et al. (2022). Professional midwifery advocates: delivering restorative clinical supervision. *Nursing Times* 118 (2): 26–28.

Flack, L. and Abdulmohdi, N. (2023). Designing and delivering a professional nurse advocate training module. *Nursing Times* 119: 11.

FONS (2023). *Resilience Based Clinical Supervision: A Facilitator Companion*, 2e. University of Nottingham.

Gilbert, P. (2010). *The Compassionate Mind*. London: Constable and Robinson.

Greenberg, N. and Tracy, D. (2020). What healthcare leaders need to do to protect the psychological well-being of frontline staff in the COVID-19 pandemic. *BMJ Leader* 4: 101–102. https://doi.org/10.1136/leader-2020-000273.

Konopka, C.L., Adaime, M.B., and Mosele, P.H. (2015). Active teaching and learning methodologies: some considerations. *Creative Education* 6 (14): 1536–1545.

Lees-Deutsch, L., Kneafsey, R., Palmer, S., and Wilde, L. (2025). *Supervision, Support and Advocacy for Improvement in Nursing: A Study to Understand the Impact that PNAs Have on Patient Outcomes and Patient Experience, through Quality Improvement Projects they Lead*. Coventry University. ISBN: 978-1-84600-13201 https://doi.org/10.18552/CHC/2025/0005.

NHS England (2017). *A-EQUIP A Model of Clinical Midwifery Supervision*. London: NHS England.

NHS England (2022). Professional nurse advocate. http://www.england.nhs.uk/nursingmidwifery/delivering-the-nhs-ltp/professional-nurse-advocate (accessed 10 October 2024).

NHS England (2023). Professional nurse advocate. https://www.england.nhs.uk/long-read/pna-equip-model-a-model-of-clinical-supervision-for-nurses (accessed 15 November 2024).

NHS England (2024). NHS standard contract 2025/26 general conditions (full length). https://www.england.nhs.uk/wp-content/uploads/2025/04/04-full-length-general-conditions-2526-med-opt-mc.pdf (accessed 1 August 2024).

Nursing Midwifery Council (2018). The code (accessed 5 January 2025).

Pettit, A., Stephen, R., and Nettleton, R. (2015). *Developing Resilience in the Workforce: A Health Visiting Framework Guide for Employers, Managers and Team Leaders*. London: Institute of Health Visiting, Health Education England and the Department of Health.

Royal College of Nursing (2021). *Principles of Nursing Practice*. The Royal College of Nursing.

Royal College of Nursing (2023). Professional nurse advocate standards for education and training programmes and modules. `www.rcn.org.uk/Professional-Development/publications/professional-nurse-advocate-standards-uk` pub-010-854 (accessed 15 November 2024).

Smith, J. (2021). *Nurturing Maternity Staff: How to Tackle Trauma, Stress and Burnout to Create a Positive Working Culture in the NHS*. Pinter & Martin.

Stovall, M., Hansen, L., and van Ryn, M. (2020). A critical review: moral injury in nurses in the aftermath of a patient safety incident. *Journal of Nursing Scholarship* 52 (3): 320–328. `https://doi.org/10.1111/jnu.12551`. Epub 2020 Mar 28. PMID: 32222036.

The King's Fund (2020) The Courage of Compassion: Supporting Nurses and Midwives to Deliver High-quality Care.

Wallbank, S. and Woods, G. (2012). A healthier health visiting workforce: findings from the restorative supervision programme. *Community Practitioner* 85 (11): 20–23.

CHAPTER 5

Developing Restorative Supervision in the PNA Role

Adele Parsons

RN, ACP, QN, Senior Lecturer, University of Lincoln, UK

INTRODUCTION

The aim of this chapter is to provide a comprehensive and accessible introduction to restorative clinical supervision (RCS) for Professional Nurse Advocates (PNAs). It seeks to clarify the principles underpinning RCS, its distinctive contribution in comparison with other forms of professional support, and its significance for contemporary nursing practice. The chapter is intended to build both theoretical understanding and practical confidence by outlining approaches, techniques and strategies relevant to supervisors and supervisees alike. In addition, examples drawn from clinical contexts will be used to demonstrate how RCS operates in practice and how it can contribute to professional well-being, resilience, and the enhancement of nursing practice. In doing so, the chapter aims to ensure that RCS is presented as both an understandable and applicable process that supports personal and professional development.

How to Use this Chapter

You can get the most out of this chapter in a few different ways. It's helpful to read it once from start to finish to get the big picture and understand how all the ideas fit together, or you may prefer to bookmark elements, or dip in and out.

For PNAs: You can use the *Top Tips* and *Notes* sections as points to guide your thinking before or after a supervision session, helping you stay focused and reflective. The RCS Case Studies offer real-world examples that show how the concepts play out in everyday nursing practice, making the theory more relatable and applicable. The RCS structure works well as a checklist, supporting your preparation and ensuring that all essential elements of supervision are covered. The *RCS Toolbox* provides practical resources you can draw on during sessions and revisit afterwards to reinforce learning. Finally, the networking section at the end of the chapter suggests useful contacts and ongoing resources to help sustain your role and build a supportive professional community.

For Supervisees: This chapter is designed to help you prepare for and reflect on your own supervision experiences. The *Top Tips* offer quick, practical pointers to help you get the most out of each session, while the *Notes* highlight important messages throughout the text to support your learning. Case Studies show how others have used the RCS approach in practice, giving you real-life examples to relate to. Activities are included for you to pause and reflect on your own experiences. Using the RCS structure as a prompt will help to guide your thinking and preparation to engage in meaningful reflection. You might also find the *RCS Toolbox* and networking section helpful for building your confidence, accessing useful resources, and strengthening your professional support system.

BACKGROUND AND CONTEXT

The 2024 NHS Staff Survey highlighted that workforce well-being remains under significant pressure, with over two in five staff (41.6%) reporting feeling unwell due to work-related stress – a figure virtually unchanged from the previous year (NHS England, 2025). Stress, anxiety, depression and other psychiatric illnesses remain the single most common cause of sickness absence across the NHS, accounting for more than a quarter of all days lost (NHS Digital 2024). Analysis by the Nuffield Trust (2025) identified that the proportion of staff reporting feeling unwell as a result of work-related stress remains worryingly high and there is a risk this is being normalised. For nurses specifically, the Royal College of Nursing (2024) reported that stress-related absences rose from 21.0% in 2022 to 24.3% in 2023, equating to nearly seven million working days lost in a single year. Although reports of burnout have eased slightly since the peak of the pandemic, nearly a third of NHS staff still describe feeling burned out 'often' or 'always', underscoring the scale and persistence of the well-being crisis in the nursing workforce (The King's Fund 2025).

Against this backdrop, the role of the PNA and the use of RCS have become increasingly important. PNAs, introduced nationally in England in 2021, are trained to provide structured supportive supervision using the Advocating for Education and Quality Improvement (A-EQUIP) model with a strong restorative focus (NHSE 2022). This enables nurses and other staff to reflect on their experiences in a psychologically safe space, fostering resilience and reducing the emotional burden of practice. By embedding RCS into everyday professional culture, PNAs play a key role in addressing the drivers of stress and burnout that are so clearly reflected in the national survey data (Griffiths 2022).

The evidence base for RCS demonstrates tangible benefits for staff and organisations, providing a strategy to mitigate workplace stress associated with a 43% reduction in burnout and 62% reduction in stress levels among participants (Wallbank and Woods 2012). Wider studies of restorative group supervision have similarly shown increases in compassion satisfaction, reductions in sickness absence and strengthened emotional resilience (Wallbank and Hatton 2011). These findings position RCS not only as a supportive intervention but also as a strategic workforce investment, with the potential to reduce attrition, improve patient care and sustain the long-term health of the NHS workforce (RCN 2022).

BRIEF HISTORY OF CLINICAL SUPERVISION IN NURSING

Clinical supervision has been part of nursing practice in various forms for over 30 years (Masamha et al. 2022). In the 1990s, Butterworth and Fougier (1992) described it as 'a process that promoted personal and professional development within a supportive relationship'. This definition emphasised the dual purpose of supervision: supporting both professional growth and individual well-being. In 1998, the Department of Health further endorsed clinical supervision in its white paper, marking it as a formal component of nursing practice.

Despite its long history, clinical supervision in nursing was often perceived as informal peer support rather than a structured process. More formal supervisory frameworks were sometimes seen as authoritarian or punitive, limiting their uptake and impact (Butterworth and Fougier 1992). Exceptions included midwifery, health visiting and district nursing, while fields such as social work and clinical psychology had long recognised supervision as a protective factor against burnout and work-related stress (Hill 1989; Copp 1988). In the national evaluation of PNA implementation, Lees-Deutsch et al. (2025) found that nurses who were not aware of formal frameworks thought RCS was a 'good addition' and those who were aware of formal frameworks felt RCS was distinctive and different.

Move to a Restorative Model of Supervision

The emotional labour inherent in nursing has long been recognised as a significant contributor to stress, compassion fatigue and burnout (Hochschild 1983; Figley 1995). Challenges, which existed prior to the pandemic, were intensified during COVID-19, highlighting the need for supervision that explicitly prioritised emotional support and restoration. Traditional models often focused primarily on performance or learning, with limited attention to the psychological impact of caregiving. RCS was developed to address this gap, providing structured, reflective spaces for staff to process the emotional demands of their work, build resilience and maintain well-being.

Table illustrates shift to RCS

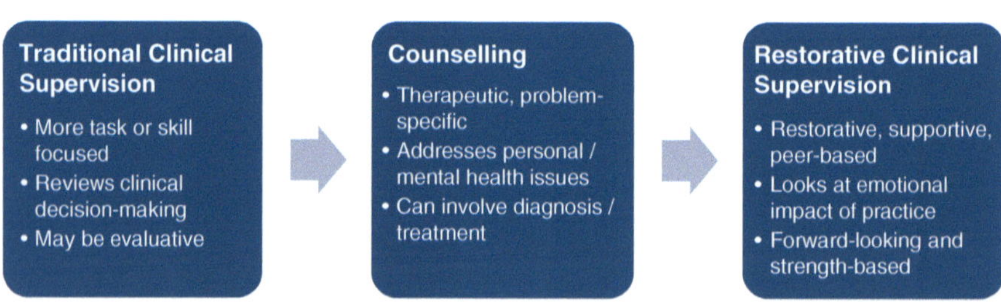

RCS focuses on emotional and psychological support for staff. It was developed from the work of Wallbank and Robertson (2008), who explored how nurses, midwives and doctors in maternity care managed the emotional labour of miscarriage, stillbirth and loss. Their research highlighted the cost of caregiving on staff well-being and the need for structured emotional support. The first pilot study in 2009, a small randomised controlled trial, showed that staff receiving RCS reported reduced stress, lower burnout, increased compassion satisfaction and improved compassion fatigue scores, while those in the control group showed no change. Subsequent studies with larger groups of community doctors, nurses and social workers found that resilience-based supervision consistently reduced burnout by 43% and stress by 62% (Wallbank and Woods 2012).

At its core, RCS provides structured, reflective supervision that is supportive, validating, and restorative, integrating principles from psychology, emotional intelligence and trauma-informed practice. The model is built around four key elements and is often cited as a gold standard for emotionally intelligent and compassionate supervision:

1. **Emotional Processing:** Creating safe spaces for staff to explore and validate feelings about challenging or distressing situations.
2. **Resilience Building:** Reflecting on personal strengths and coping strategies to foster long-term emotional resilience.
3. **Restorative Dialogue:** Restoring a sense of purpose, value and connection with work, aligned with organisational values and promoting compassion and peer support.
4. **Structured Supervision:** Delivered in 1:1 or group settings, with regular, facilitated sessions to maintain consistency and impact (Wallbank and Hatton 2011).

Pettit and Stephen (2015) further validated RCS as a preventative and supportive intervention, demonstrating reductions in stress, burnout and emotional exhaustion, while improving resilience, job satisfaction and professional engagement.

> **Note:** Evidence consistently shows creating space for staff to reflect, feel heard and explore challenges builds resilience and problem-solving skills – benefiting both individuals and the wider organisation.

Role of Professional Nurse Advocates

The introduction of PNAs in England through the A-EQUIP model formalised the delivery of RCS across the nursing workforce (NHS England 2021). The recent national evaluation of the PNA programme (Lees-Deutsch et al. 2025) highlights its substantial impact, including improvements in nurse empowerment, psychological well-being and job satisfaction. Since implementation, the programme has delivered over 78,000 RCS sessions, nearly 50,000 career conversations and more than 2500 quality improvement projects. Key factors for success included safe, structured spaces, adequate time for supervision and organisational commitment. Challenges such as time pressures and the need for sustained institutional support were also noted, underscoring that effective implementation requires both individual and systemic engagement.

These findings underscore the value of PNAs in embedding RCS into everyday practice, providing both emotional support and professional development, while highlighting the practical considerations essential for sustaining the programme's impact.

Overall, both historical and contemporary evidence illustrates the critical importance of RCS in supporting the emotional and professional well-being of nursing staff. Pettit and Stephen (2015) and the national PNA evaluation (Lees-Deutsch et al. 2025) consistently demonstrate that RCS reduces stress and burnout, enhances resilience and improves professional engagement. By providing staff with opportunities to reflect, be heard and explore the emotional challenges of their roles, RCS fosters psychological safety, professional growth and improved patient care outcomes.

Embedding RCS within the nursing workforce aligns with the NHS People Promise, which commits to valuing, supporting and empowering staff, as well as the long-term goals outlined in the NHS Long Term Plan and NHS People Plan workforce strategy, both of which prioritise staff well-being as fundamental to high-quality, sustainable care (NHS England, 2025; NHS England 2020). Given the ongoing pressures highlighted in national staff surveys – including persistent stress, burnout and mental health-related absence – it is clear that interventions such as RCS should be considered a strategic priority. Its implementation through PNAs illustrates how structured, restorative supervision can both meet these commitments and support workforce sustainability, while also recognising the practical need for organisational commitment and protected time to ensure lasting impact.

UNDERSTANDING EMOTIONS

Understanding how emotions function – what they are, how they arise, and their physiological impact – is essential in the context of RCS. Emotions are compelling because they are rooted in complex biological processes that influence cognition, behaviour and interpersonal interactions (Fox 2008). The fight-or-flight response, for example, is an evolutionary mechanism designed to protect us from physical threats (Cannon 1929). While the nature of threats in modern clinical environments has changed, our bodies still respond with the same physiological intensity. This can lead to automatic reactions that may be unhelpful or even counterproductive in professional settings. Each emotion carries a distinct biological signature, influencing heart rate, hormone levels and neural activity. Recognising these responses allows PNAs and nurses to better understand the emotional landscape of supervision and respond with greater awareness and regulation.

- **With Fear**: Circuits in the brain's emotional centre trigger a flood of hormones that put us on high alert, so we can focus our attention on the perceived threat. Blood is redirected to the large skeletal muscles such as the legs, making it easier for us to run; the face blanches as blood is redirected leading to the expression *your blood runs cold*.
- **With Anger:** We experience a rush of hormones such as adrenaline that generates a pulse of energy strong enough for us to jump into action; blood flows to the hands making it easier to grab a weapon or strike out at an enemy.
- **Sadness:** When we are sad the body's metabolism slows, focus becomes more introspective and we might see a drop in energy and enthusiasm. Researchers think that this loss of energy may have been a protective factor and kept our ancestors closer to home when they were vulnerable – where they were safer and could be protected.
- **In Happiness:** Increased activity means that feelings of negativity and worrisome thoughts are suppressed. This creates a rest or peacefulness for the brain where it can recover from more upsetting emotions. This recovery space is calming and can lead to a natural desire to return to the task that brings about this feeling – especially important when managing stress or preventing burnout.

The biological basis for many emotional responses is rooted in primitive brain structures designed for survival (Ekman 1999). Unlike our ancestors, we have developed the capacity to regulate these emotions; we do not act on impulse when angry or retreat when sad. Emotional regulation is a learned skill, enabling us to respond thoughtfully rather than react instinctively.

Brain Structures and Emotional Response

Understanding how different parts of the brain contribute to emotional and stress responses is essential in RCS. Each region plays a distinct role in how we react, regulate and reflect.

- **Reptilian Brain (Brainstem):** The brainstem, the most primitive part of the brain, regulates essential life functions such as heart rate, breathing and body temperature. It operates automatically and consistently, prioritising survival. While it can be temporarily overridden by higher brain functions (e.g. holding your breath), it ultimately regains control to maintain homeostasis.

- **Limbic Brain (Emotional Brain):** The limbic system processes emotions, memory and motivation. Structures like the amygdala trigger rapid, unconscious responses to perceived threats – such as the fight-or-flight reaction. Although these responses are automatic, the frontal lobes can provide rational context, allowing for more measured reactions. Techniques like deep breathing, mindfulness and social connection help downregulate this stress response.

- **Neocortex (Thinking Brain):** The neocortex governs higher order functions including reasoning, language and conscious thought. It enables us to override automatic emotional reactions and respond with reflection and intention – critical skills in emotionally charged environments like clinical supervision. (MacLean 1990)

Understanding the neurobiology of stress is essential for supervisors delivering RCS. Stress triggers chemical responses – such as the release of cortisol – that affect the body at a cellular level, with prolonged exposure linked to damage in brain structures like the hippocampus, contributing to symptoms such as brain fog and impaired decision-making (Talbot 2007; Wallbank and Robertson 2008). The amygdala, responsible for processing emotions like anxiety and frustration, can overwhelm the neocortex under pressure, reducing our capacity for rational thought. Kahneman (2011) describes this shift as a dominance of Type 1 thinking – fast, automatic and emotionally driven – over Type 2 thinking, which is slower and reflective.

> **TOP TIP**
>
> If a supervisee is reacting from a heightened emotional state, pause and create space for calm reflection – this helps shift the conversation towards clearer, more considered thinking.

Wallbank (2016) emphasises that a key underpinning theory of the restorative resilience model is the understanding that it is our response to the stressor – not the stressor itself – that determines its impact. When stress is unmanaged, it can manifest in workplace behaviours such as lateness, absence, low morale, relationship difficulties, reduced productivity, avoidance of emotional involvement, lack of motivation, feeling overwhelmed, reluctance to engage, difficulty in decision-making and, ultimately, burnout and compassion fatigue (Wallbank 2010). For PNAs, this understanding is vital; by recognising the physiological and psychological effects of stress, supervisors can develop strategies to support emotional regulation, foster resilience and promote reflective and reflexive practice. Identifying triggers, processing emotional responses and implementing coping strategies are key components of effective supervision and professional well-being.

ACTIVITY

How do you react to stress? What are your triggers?

What are those early warning signs: irritation? withdrawal?

If you don't know, perhaps ask those close to you

What words or behaviours trigger extreme responses at work?

What can you do to prevent this from happening?

By recognising what triggers our emotional responses and how we typically react, we can begin to manage unhelpful patterns and develop more constructive ways of responding.

Emotional Labour in Nursing

Emotional labour, a concept introduced by Arlie Hochschild in The Managed Heart (1983), refers to the effort required to manage your own emotions to meet the expectations of your role. In nursing, this often means displaying patience, empathy, or calmness even when your internal feelings are very different – like remaining composed with an aggressive patient or supporting a grieving family while managing your own emotions.

Hochschild identified two ways this 'hard emotional work' can be done:

- **Deep Acting:** Actively working to change your internal feelings so they align with what is required. Over time, this can be protective for well-being because your emotions and your role are more aligned.
- **Surface Acting:** Simply faking the expected emotion without changing how you feel inside. While easier in the short term, surface acting is draining and can affect long-term well-being.

Emotional labour is a demanding and often invisible aspect of caring work, yet it plays a central role in shaping both patient experience and staff well-being. Its cumulative nature means that, if left unacknowledged, it can impact resilience over time. Actively recognising and reflecting on your emotional responses is key to managing emotional labour effectively. While deep acting involves genuinely aligning your emotions with your professional role, surface acting requires you to mask or fake them – something that can take a toll if sustained. Taking time to reflect on these emotional strategies helps protect well-being and supports a more sustainable approach to care.

1:1 RCS Unplanned

A colleague approached me informally expressing emotional exhaustion and disconnection from role and considering a gap year or resignation as no longer able to see joy or fulfilment in her role.

Offered to sit down, away from the ward environment, in psychologically safe space and used open-ended questions to explore emotional state, coping strategies and potential sources of burnout (Beinart et al. 2016; Johnson et al. 2020; West et al. 2020).

Found it quite a powerful space for both of us, everyone thought this individual was so confident and never verbalised these feelings before. Lainidi et al. (2025) found evidence to support the link between emotional exhaustion and employee silence, with a high correlation between employee silence and burnout. Suppression of emotions is seen as a maladaptive approach that can have longer term impacts (Brockman et al. 2016).

THE SUPERVISOR IN RESTORATIVE CLINICAL SUPERVISION

Supervisors engaging in RCS must recognise the emotional demands of the role and prepare accordingly. Entering a supervision session should be approached with the same diligence as a personal risk assessment. This involves thoughtful reflection on several key considerations, consider:

Questions to Consider Before Undertaking RCS

Am I the most appropriate person to facilitate this session?

Am I prepared?

What emotional or professional themes might arise and can I remain impartial throughout?

Is RCS the most suitable approach for this context and is it likely to be beneficial?

Are the supervisees prepared – are they in the right mental and emotional space to engage meaningfully? Would this session work better as a 1:1 or 1:group?

Clarifying the purpose of the session is essential: Are we seeking solutions, exploring emotional responses or focusing on a particular issue? Supervisors must also anticipate and plan for the management of strong emotions, particularly in group settings where diverse personalities may influence dynamics. Effective facilitation requires ensuring all voices are heard, balancing contributions and maintaining psychological safety. Finally, supervisors should consider how the session will be brought to a close and what resources or follow-up support may be required. This reflective preparation not only safeguards the well-being of the supervisees but also supports the supervisor in maintaining professional boundaries and emotional resilience.

TOP TIP

Think of this self-check-in as fitting your own oxygen mask before assisting others, supervisors must prioritise their own emotional well-being to effectively support their supervisee.

PNAs must also reflect on their proximity to the supervisee – professionally, personally or hierarchically – as this can influence the dynamics of the session. In some cases, it may be beneficial to offer the option of engaging with a PNA who is less familiar to the nurse. This can help mitigate concerns around vulnerability, reluctance to disclose or perceived judgement. Confidentiality and trust are foundational to effective restorative supervision and creating conditions that support openness is essential. PNAs should consider whether their relationship with the supervisee might inhibit honest reflection and, where appropriate, facilitate access to alternative supervision arrangements that better support psychological safety (Rouse 2019).

1:1 Supervision–supervisor Reflection

As a new nurse providing RCS, I initially felt anxious about whether I had the skills to support colleagues effectively. Reading about liminal spaces (Liedgren et al. 2023) helped me recognise that entering this new role

(continued)

(continued)

might feel unfamiliar and uncertain, but that this was part of the process. During practice, I realised that my role was not to provide all the answers but to create a supportive space where others could reflect and reach their own conclusions. This aligned with the NMC Code (2018), particularly around professionalism, trust and collaboration. By focusing on these values, I was able to feel more confident and I found it very rewarding to see how I had helped a colleague through reflection.

Emotional Intelligence

Emotional intelligence (EI) is a key skill for supervisors. Goleman (2000) describes four areas of EI: self-awareness, self-management, social awareness and relationship management. These skills help supervisors handle sensitive conversations, create a safe space and respond with empathy. In nursing, EI has been linked to compassionate care and stronger team relationships (Carragher and Gormley 2017). In RCS, both supervisor and supervisee can use EI to notice and understand emotions as they arise in the session. This might involve recognising what they are feeling, exploring where those feelings come from, and thinking together about how to respond in a positive way. By practising this, supervisees learn not only to manage their own emotions but also to respond more constructively in challenging clinical situations. Over time, this builds resilience, improves communication and strengthens the supportive nature of the supervisory relationship.

ACTIVITY: CHECKING IN WITH YOUR EMOTIONS

Think about a common situation at work that triggers a strong emotional response

What kind of situation usually brings up strong emotions?

How do you typically feel and react in this situation?

What effect does this response have on you, your practice and others?

How could I use this emotion in a constructive way or respond differently next time?

One small action I will try when this situation comes up again is...

Leadership

The PNA is fundamentally a leadership role, requiring individuals to guide, support and influence others through restorative approaches. Chapter 4 offers a deeper exploration of leadership. When delivering RCS PNAs must embody leadership qualities that align with the ethos of the model – creating psychologically safe environments, fostering emotional resilience and enabling reflective practice. Leadership in this context is not about authority, but about relational presence, EI and skilled facilitation.

Transformational and authentic leadership styles are particularly effective in RCS. These approaches are characterised by transparency, integrity and a focus on relationships, enabling supervisors to lead with purpose while empowering supervisees to explore their experiences openly (Martin and Milne 2018). The tandem model of supervision exemplifies this balance, positioning the supervisor as both guide and collaborator. Self-awareness is also a critical leadership attribute; supervisors must reflect on their own values, biases and behaviours to avoid blind spots and foster mutual respect (Lockwood 2024).

Compassionate leadership, as defined by West and Chowla (2017), offers a particularly relevant framework for RCS. It involves attending, understanding, empathising and helping – principles that closely mirror the restorative model. In clinical supervision, this means being present with the supervisee, listening actively, and responding with empathy and support. Compassion and empathy are not optional; they are essential in creating a space where supervisees can explore challenges, reduce emotional burden, and reconnect with their professional purpose. Wallbank (2013) found that restorative supervision significantly reduced burnout and increased compassion satisfaction among nurses, illuminating the value of emotionally intelligent leadership.

PNAs must also balance compassion with boundaries. RCS can be emotionally demanding, and supervisors must prioritise their own well-being – akin to fitting their own oxygen mask before assisting others. This includes recognising emotional fatigue, when engaging in supervision, and accessing their own support systems when needed. Ultimately, leadership in RCS requires the ability to listen deeply, respond thoughtfully, and create conditions where reflection leads to growth. In doing so, supervisors not only support individual well-being but contribute to a culture of compassion, safety, and resilience across the organisation.

Active Listening

Active listening is a cornerstone of effective RCS, enabling supervisors to create a psychologically safe space where supervisees feel genuinely heard, understood and valued. Within the PNA framework, active listening is not merely a communication technique but a therapeutic tool that facilitates emotional processing, reflective thinking and resilience building. Supervisors help staff to reflect on their experiences, to inform future decision-making (Applewhite et al. 2022). This approach is particularly impactful in high-pressure clinical environments, where nurses often feel unseen or overwhelmed. Research from Great Ormond Street Hospital found that RCS helped nurses harness their voice, especially those experiencing low confidence or burnout, by offering a space for reflection and validation (Houlihan et al. 2022). Supervisors must develop skills in attentive silence, paraphrasing, emotional attunement and non-verbal responsiveness to facilitate this process. The national evaluation of the PNA programme further supports this, highlighting that nurses who received RCS reported increased psychological empowerment and a renewed sense of professional purpose (Lees-Deutsch et al. 2025). Thus, active listening within RCS is not passive – it is an intentional, skilled practice that underpins the restorative function of supervision and contributes meaningfully to workforce well-being and retention.

Supervisors must engage in continuous professional development to maintain the quality and impact of RCS. While the PNA programme provides a robust foundation for practice, ongoing development in supervision models, feedback techniques and leadership is essential. Skills in restorative supervision are akin to developing a new muscle – initially unfamiliar, requiring regular use and strengthened through consistent practice. Given the emotional complexity of RCS, particularly when navigating sensitive or distressing content, supervisors must remain confident and competent in their approach. The national evaluation of the PNA programme identified that 18% of PNAs had yet to undertake RCS, reflected in comments around not using skills (Lees-Deutsch et al. 2023). Regular engagement not only sustains individual capability but also contributes to the broader organisational culture of support and psychological safety.

> **Note:** The A in Professional Nurse Advocate stands for Advocacy: This means helping colleagues find their own way through reflection, empowering others to navigate their own challenges, not fixing or providing solutions for them.

THE SUPERVISEE IN RESTORATIVE CLINICAL SUPERVISION

RCS offers healthcare professionals a vital space to reflect, recharge and realign, while the supervisor facilitates the process, the supervisee's engagement is equally essential. Knowing how to prepare, participate and reflect can transform supervision into a deeply restorative and empowering experience.

To get the most out of RCS, supervisees are encouraged to approach sessions with openness, curiosity and a willingness to reflect. The most meaningful sessions often emerge when supervisees:

- **Engage Actively**: Share thoughts, feelings, and experiences honestly – even if they feel messy or unresolved.
- **Set Intentions:** Consider what you hope to gain – clarity, emotional release, problem-solving or simply space to be heard.
- **Trust the Process**: Even if the session feels slow, emotional or uncertain, these are often signs of deep reflection and growth.

Preparation can help maximise the value of each session. Supervisees might find it helpful to:

- **Reflect on Recent Experiences:** What has challenged or uplifted you? What's been emotionally significant?
- **Identify Themes**: Are there recurring patterns in your work or emotions that you'd like to explore?
- **Be Honest:** If something feels difficult to talk about, name that feeling – it's a powerful starting point.
- **Bring Prompts:** Notes, reflective journals, feedback or patient stories can help guide the conversation.
- **Don't Over-prepare**: Sometimes the most valuable insights come from spontaneous reflection.

Arriving a few minutes early, taking a breath and mentally transitioning into the reflective space can also help settle into the session.

What to Expect from RCS

Quality supervision should feel:

- **Non-judgemental**: You are not being assessed or evaluated.
- **Safe:** Confidentiality and psychological safety are paramount.

- **Unhurried:** There is time to think, feel and speak without pressure.
- **Supportive:** Your supervisor is there to listen, guide and hold space.

You may experience silence, emotion or uncertainty – and that's okay. These are often signs of deep processing and should be welcomed rather than avoided.

If you're new to RCS, the process may feel unfamiliar. It's common to feel unsure about what to say or how to 'do it right'. Supervisors can help by normalising these feelings and gently guiding the conversation. Over time, trust builds, and the process becomes more natural.

Practical tips for settling in:

- **Start Small**: Share a recent moment that stood out, even if it seems minor.
- **Use Metaphors**: If emotions are hard to name, describe them as weather, colours or sensations.
- **Ask Questions**: 'Is this a good topic for supervision?' or 'Can we explore this together?' are great ways to open dialogue.

After supervision, take a moment to note what stood out and how you feel – good supervision often brings a sense of clarity and a lighter emotional load, as highlighted in the experiences shared by nurses in the clinical supervision process (Lees-Deutsch et al. 2025).

RCS Example from Practice

A colleague who worked in the same department in a junior role, she was perceived by the whole of the team negatively as someone who complained regularly, this could be particularly disruptive to new staff or students on placement. This member of staff approached me for a 1:1 supervision session and honestly at that first session pretty much all I did was listen, there was a lot of venting and frustration. At the end of the session we agreed 2 points with easy practical solutions that could be implemented easily. A couple of months later the staff member approached me for another supervision session and shared how powerful the first session had been, she realised that some things couldn't be changed but recognised the changes we had made and the positive impact. For most of the session she vented, I listened. This pattern continued and, over time I recognised 2 things: (i). She just needed a safe space to talk things out, and by venting in a controlled way her daily frustrations were minimised. (ii). The way the rest of the team viewed this member of staff changed, she was no longer seen in a negative light, the suggestions she made that were acted on benefitted everyone and she was credited with suggesting the changes that worked.

For this colleague, 1:1 supervision created a psychologically safe space for reflection and emotional release. Rather than focusing on blame, the sessions encouraged honest dialogue and surfaced deeper concerns – such as anxiety around change or feelings of being unheard and undervalued. Supervision became a meaningful outlet to explore emotional responses and gain insight into personal and professional experiences. As trust grew, so did team cohesion. The supervisee felt empowered to speak openly, and previously negative comments that had been affecting the wider team diminished significantly. With a dedicated space to offload and reflect, the nurse reported feeling a stronger sense of belonging, and described the sessions as both motivating and fulfilling.

STRUCTURING RCS

RCS can be undertaken as an ad hoc intervention – through corridor conversations, water cooler moments or opportunistic team check-ins during handover periods. However, while these informal interactions are valuable, RCS is most effective when embedded as a regular, structured practice within a teams' routine.

Nurses need to 'settle in' to supervision; (see image below) the national evaluation (Lees-Deutsch et al. 2025) identified many nurses demonstrated a cautious approach to supervision with uncertainty, self-doubt and for some self-consciousness. A need to understand the process and in some cases build trust in this relationship may take time and multiple sessions. RCS is an ongoing process that is fundamentally an investment in building a trusting relationship between a supervisor and a supervisee. Unlike traditional, more task-focused supervision, the restorative approach prioritises the supervisee's emotional well-being, providing a consistent 'thinking space' to reflect on the emotional impact of their work. This relational investment is what makes the process effective in building staff resilience and mitigating burnout.

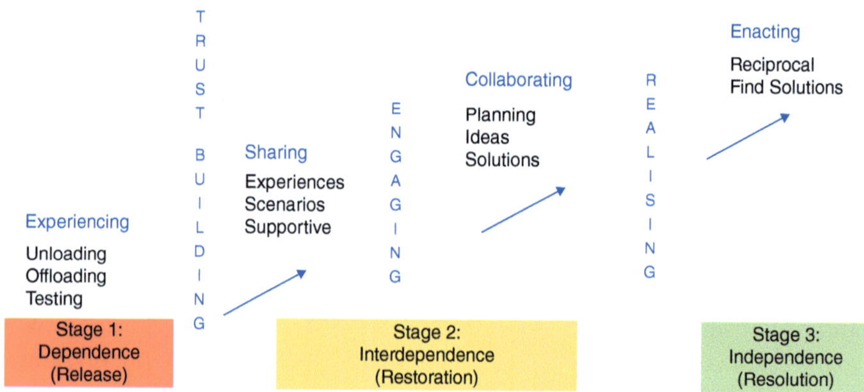

Image National Evaluation of PNA Programme (Lees-Deutsch et al., 2023, p78).
Source: Coventry University, 2023 / with permission of Coventry University

Evidence from the National Evaluation Report of the PNA in England supports the view of RCS as a developmental process that unfolds in three stages, moving from dependence to independence (Lees-Deutsch et al. 2025). In the first stage, Release (dependence), nurses engage in unloading, offloading, and testing feelings within a safe environment, which creates the foundation of trust and psychological safety. The second stage, Restoration (interdependence), is characterised by sharing experiences, mutual support and moving towards collective planning and problem-solving. Finally, the third stage, Realisation (independence), involves reciprocity, solution finding, and increased professional confidence, enabling staff to feel empowered and resilient. Importantly, RCS should be viewed as an ongoing process that requires time to develop relationships; only when trust and deeper connections are established can the higher achievements of innovation, quality improvement and cultural change be realised. In this sense, RCS not only restores individual well-being but also provides a foundation for professional growth and systemic improvement (Lees-Deutsch et al. 2025).

Group Supervision

For RCS to be sustainable within organisations, it may not always be feasible to offer individual one-to-one sessions. Group supervision, therefore, presents a valuable alternative. In professions where practitioners often work in isolation – even within busy environments – group sessions offer a space for reconnection and shared reflection. Wallbank (2013) observed that these sessions allow participants to explore ideas collaboratively, normalise emotional responses, and collectively examine workplace pressures. This shared understanding can foster innovative solutions and enhance resilience. Importantly, Wallbank found that group restorative experiences not only complemented individual sessions but also provided an efficient and effective means of delivering the restorative model at scale, benefiting both individuals and the wider organisation. Subsequent evaluations, such as Beckwith (2022), and findings from the national PNA programme (Lees-Deutsch et al. 2023), echoed this sentiment, with nurses valuing group supervision as a space for peer discussion and idea sharing. However, group supervision is not without its challenges. Supervisors must skilfully navigate group dynamics, ensuring that both dominant and quieter voices are heard. As Valentino et al. (2016) notes, the supervisor's role is to lead without dominating, offering appropriate and constructive feedback while facilitating inclusive dialogue. This requires a high level of interpersonal skill and sensitivity to ensure that all participants feel safe, valued, and able to contribute meaningfully.

Considerations for Group Supervision

Clarify the Purpose

- Define the aim of the session: reflection, emotional support, problem-solving or team cohesion.
- Who do you expect to attend, are there any key individuals who should attend and do you need to consider shift patterns.
- Share the purpose with participants in advance to set expectations and allow them to prepare.

Select an Appropriate Environment

- Select a space with adequate capacity.
- Choose a quiet, neutral space that supports confidentiality and comfort.
- Arrange seating in a circle or semicircle to encourage openness and equality.

(continued)

(continued)

Plan the Structure

- Use a consistent format (e.g. check-in, reflective discussion and summary).
- Allow time for each participant to speak but remain flexible to group needs.
- Use inclusive facilitation techniques to invite quieter members to contribute: Would you like to add anything?
- Gently manage dominant voices to ensure balance.
- Be attuned to emotional shifts – pause if needed, validate feelings.

Prepare Yourself

- Reflect on your own emotional state and readiness to facilitate.
- Consider group dynamics – are there dominant voices that may need to be managed? How will you do this? Are there quieter members or unresolved tensions?

Set Ground Rules

- Co-create agreements around confidentiality, respect and participation.
- Reinforce that supervision is a non-judgemental space.

Have Resources Ready

- Bring reflective prompts, well-being tools, or signposting materials.
- Know where to refer individuals if deeper support is needed.

Close with Intention

- Summarise key reflections or themes.
- End with a well-being check or a forward-looking question: 'What will you take away from today?'

Reflect Afterwards

- Take time to debrief yourself – what went well and what could be improved?
- Consider peer supervision or journaling to support your own development.

Reflection on Group RCS

Facilitating a group RCS session brought its own complexities. Each participant came with their own perspective, and not everyone felt equally comfortable with the restorative approach. Some joined out of a sense of duty to their colleagues rather than personal preference, which reminded me of the influence of group dynamics and subtle biases, like confirmation bias.

I came to understand that part of my role was to ensure that quieter voices had space to be heard, without forcing participation. As Scanlon and Hart (2024) notes, group RCS can stir a range of dynamics that require sensitive facilitation – being present to guide the conversation without dominating it. Interestingly, some participants found value simply by listening, without speaking. One staff member shared, 'I thought asking for help would be seen as weakness', which opened up a powerful discussion about vulnerability as a strength.

Throughout the session, I paid close attention to non-verbal cues and noticed who hadn't spoken. At the end, I invited each person to share – if they wished – whether the session had helped and in what way. We also used the normative function to explore relevant policies and protocols, which led to identifying gaps in training and support around conflict management.

TOP TIP

Group supervision can be tricky to manage, especially when ensuring everyone has a chance to contribute. Try using a simple 'queue system': participants raise their hand to speak, then hold up one finger if they are first in line, two fingers if they are second, and so on. This keeps track of the order fairly, reduces bias and makes sure all voices are heard.

RCS Exemplar Group Supervision

The session was undertaken as part of consolidation following an induction period for a small group (4) of newly qualified nurses into the ICU. It became clear that many were experiencing heightened anxiety – particularly around making mistakes in such a high-stakes environment. There were some specific concerns from the group around accessing support and who they could approach as staff always appeared so busy and under pressure, the work

(continued)

(continued)

environment was different from anything they had experienced before and there were other concerns around off-duty rotas and work allocation. I felt the group had bottled up a number of issues and this gave the opportunity to voice them. It was helpful for them to be able to normalise their own concerns by realising these were shared common ground across the group. Intensive care settings often pose a steep learning curve for new practitioners and I was able to reassure them that many of their feelings were normal.

We explored Covey's (1989) Circle of Control, Influence, and Concern model. The nurses identified that while they couldn't control every aspect of theirenvironment,theycouldtakeownershipoftheirownlearning–particularly around the unit's digital systems and equipment, unfamiliarity with these tools had been affecting confidence.

I managed to catch up with the same group a few weeks later with a more structured RCS session. Through peer support and open dialogue the group began developing practical ideas of how we could better support future staff which has been adopted by the unit.

1:1 Supervision

Whilst group supervision has value and is clearly favoured by some nurses and organisations, one-to-one supervision offers a more tailored approach with a private environment for deep reflection and personal emotional exploration. One-to-one sessions allow for a focussed and individualised approach to address specific concerns or challenges where the sharing of personal emotions might be difficult in a group setting (Butterworth 2022).

When 1:1 Supervision is Most Beneficial

Addressing Personal Burnout and Stress:

For PNAs experiencing high levels of stress, anxiety or fear, a 1:1 session offers a private thinking space to process these emotions and build emotional resilience.

Processing Emotionally Demanding Work:

Complex or emotionally challenging clinical work can take a toll. 1:1 supervision allows for a focused discussion to manage these feelings, which may not be appropriate or comfortable for a group setting.

Fostering a Sense of Value and Recognition:

Individual feedback in a 1:1 session can make a PNA feel like a valued and important member of the team, empowering them to feel more resilient and prevent them from leaving their role.

Developing Self-Care Strategies:

A 1:1 session provides a tailored opportunity for a PNA to explore self-care and gain the confidence to prioritise their own well-being, a crucial aspect of building resilience in a demanding role.

Asynchronous and Synchronous Supervision

Delivering RCS to individuals' or groups' working shifts, unsocial hours, or in isolated community roles presents logistical challenges. While digital tools like Teams offer improved remote access and help bridge geographical gaps or connect dispersed teams, they also limit the ability to read non-verbal cues and assume access to confidential, quiet spaces – not always available to all staff.

Supervision doesn't need to take place in an office or clinical setting; alternative environments, such as outdoor spaces, can offer a refreshing and psychologically safe backdrop for reflection. Thoughtful use of both synchronous and asynchronous digital tools, combined with flexible approaches to location, can enhance accessibility and foster meaningful engagement.

RCS Exemplar: 1:1

Scheduled RCS with a band 5 nurse. Although a room had been booked for this scheduled supervision session I suggested we go outdoors to walk and talk as it was a nice day. Walking and talking in a natural environment provides a restorative setting for conversations that might traditionally take place in an office (McKinney 2011). This 'walk-and-talk' approach has been linked to reduced burnout in staff (van den Berg et al. 2021) and is increasingly used in coaching and supervision (Doucette 2004; McKinney 2011; Revell 2017). Being outdoors and moving side by side can lower stress, support emotional processing, stimulate reflective thinking and create a more informal, psychologically safe space that encourages openness and balanced participation.

RCS Structure

Things to consider when planning your RCS sessions

RCS Exemplar Structure	
Physical space	Plan where the activity is taking place Choose neutral, quiet spaces for supervision Ensure privacy and comfort to encourage openness Participants should be able to speak freely without interruption or being overheard Consider proximity to workplace
Outline Purpose or Aims of the session	Having a loose, non-rigid agenda can help manage the RCS experience providing structure and direction while still allowing flexibility Setting a time frame for the session is an important part of managing expectations and will help when closing the session Consider how you will monitor the time without obviously checking, consider seating, or setting an alarm allowing time to summarise, agree next steps and close When planning consider what activities participants are returning to – it may be challenging to return immediately to some settings
Psychological Space	The importance of confidentiality and a safe space, not breaching confidentiality or the NMC (2018) Code Participants will be respectful and non-judgemental Confidentiality – unless safeguarding Themes arising from supervision and any agreed actions will be recorded, no note taking Open listening – no interrupting or over speaking If group – all participants given opportunity to contribute and it should be agreed how participants indicate they wish to speak No phones
Grounding	Use grounding exercises to centre yourself and the supervisee *before* sessions Applewhite and Logan (2022) Useful tools include: body scan, mindfulness and breathing exercises
Check-in (using tools)	Tools enable a supervisor to gauge individual or group feelings; these can include visual prompts or cards. Pictures of emotional expressions can be used; however, this may be direct and challenging for some participants and the supervisor may overlay own interpretation of emotions Consider using a more abstract, less version; for example, what *is the weather like in your head today*, or images of nature – a tree in different seasons – this can open a dialogue for discussion

(Continued)

Discussion	Ask individuals what they are finding difficult or challenging Ask what is going well Recognise strengths and weaknesses Ask individually what would help to change feelings Encourage the group to plan Use active listening affirmations Repeat key phrases back to confirm understanding of key points and gain clarification If group: ensure all participants have the opportunity to speak
Useful tools to prompt discussion	Reflective prompts can be useful to foster reflection and connection: How do you feel about this, what did you do about that, how do you feel now Prompt cards can be useful if you feel there may be issues opening up Reflective models; Gibbs (1988), Johns (1995) and Rolfe et al. (2001)
Check-out and close	Summarise what has been covered Agree actions, ownership of actions and next steps Agree what will be recorded – themes Are there any useful resources for participants – agree how they will be shared and a time – frame for this Repeat emotional check-in tool Discuss self-care
Post session review	Record key themes Report any safeguarding actions Reflection; what went well – what could be improved on Do any individuals need 1:1 or are follow-up sessions needed Complete signposting identified from session within agreed time frame
Further points to consider	Body Language: Maintain open posture, avoid crossing arms and use affirming gestures like nodding Eye contact should be balanced Tone and Pace: Speak calmly and clearly, avoid rushed or overly directive tones, which can undermine psychological safety Consider access to RCS – how will participants request RCS and how frequently Some trusts have implemented an RCS passport for recipients of RCS to record their own sessions, thoughts, feelings and actions

Note: Quality supervision is an active process – it won't always feel easy, and it may sometimes feel challenging, but that's where the real growth happens.

TYPES OF RCS CONVERSATIONS

RCS offers a flexible, psychologically safe space for a range of professional conversations – from career development to emotional processing – each requiring different levels of preparation and confidence depending on the supervisee's context and needs (Lees-Deutsch et al. 2025).

Type of RCS Conversation	Purpose	Preparation Required	Confidence Considerations
Career Conversations	Explore professional identity, transitions, and future aspirations	Reflective journaling, goal-setting, CV review	May be lower during uncertainty or role change
Emotional Processing	Address distressing clinical experiences or moral injury	Emotional readiness, trust in supervisor	Often lower due to vulnerability and emotional weight
Values Clarification	Reconnect with personal and professional values	Self-reflection, values mapping	Builds over time with repeated engagement
Boundary Work	Explore emotional boundaries and role containment	Case examples, emotional mapping	May vary depending on emotional literacy
Celebratory Reflection	Acknowledge achievements and positive impact	Minimal; storytelling or feedback	Typically high; affirming and energising
Team or Role Dynamics	Navigate interpersonal or systemic challenges	Contextual awareness, feedback from peers	Depends on team culture and

Preparation for RCS conversations varies depending on the topic and emotional intensity, and supervisee confidence may fluctuate – highlighting the importance of tailoring supervision to individual needs and contexts.

RCS Exemplar 1:1 Career Conversation

Band 5 international nurse, joined the trust 6 years ago, recently applied for a number of promotions but had been unsuccessful and found this very upsetting, didn't ask for feedback after interview, found the whole experience very challenging. Feels he is being overlooked and that other staff with less experience are being promoted ahead of him, worried he is getting stuck and left behind and this has happened to a number of international nurse colleagues.

I took this discussion back to my PNA lead and we brought this subject area up at a PNA meeting (confidentially), 2 other PNAs in the Trust identified that this was something they had heard in RCS sessions. We have now created support for international nurses around applications and interview processes, so staff can be supported, we also developed a generic lunchtime webinar and altered PNA fliers to include career conversations, support with application forms and interview preparation available for all staff. There was also some work for the leadership team and conversations around Equality, Diversity, and Inclusion (EDI) and how we support our international colleagues throughout their career.

RCS Toolbox

Useful models to explore in supervision

Circles of Control, Influence and Concern in Restorative Supervision

Overview of the Tool

Based on the work of Stephen Covey (1989), the Circles of Control, Influence, and Concern model is a valuable tool for PNAs to support self-awareness and emotional resilience during supervision sessions. This model helps individuals distinguish between areas they can control, influence or are concerned about, fostering a proactive and empowered mindset.

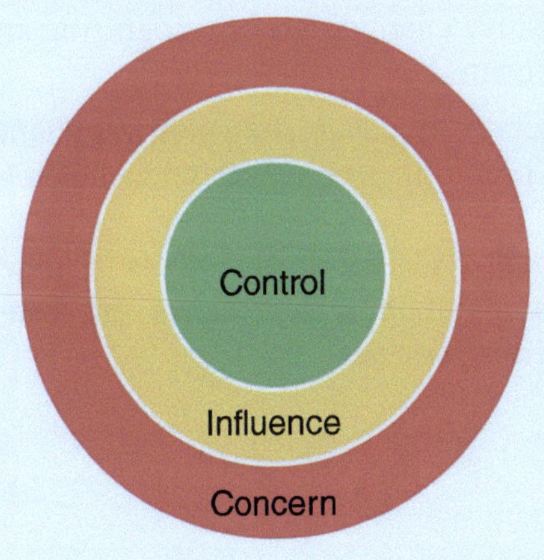

(*continued*)

(*continued*)

1. **Circle of Control:**

   This innermost circle represents aspects we have direct control over, such as our actions, responses, and attitudes. In supervision, PNAs can encourage supervisees to identify and focus on these elements, promoting a sense of agency and reducing feelings of helplessness.

2. **Circle of Influence:**

   The middle circle encompasses areas where we can exert influence, though not direct control. This includes our relationships, communication and how we engage with others. PNAs can guide supervisees to recognize and expand their influence, enhancing collaboration and support networks.

3. **Circle of Concern:**

   The outer circle includes concerns beyond our control or influence, such as systemic issues or external events. Acknowledging these concerns without dwelling on them allows supervisees to conserve emotional energy and focus on actionable areas.

Practical Application in Supervision

Identify and Reflect: Have supervisees list current challenges or stressors and categorize them into the three circles.

Discuss and Reframe: Explore how focusing on areas within the Circle of Control can lead to positive changes, while recognizing and accepting concerns outside their control.

Develop Action Plans: Collaboratively create strategies to enhance influence and manage concerns, promoting resilience and well-being.

Regular use of this model helps PNAs support supervisees in understanding their emotional responses, maintaining perspective and fostering constructive, restorative supervision sessions.

Plutchik's Wheel of Emotions

Overview of the Tool

Plutchik's Wheel of Emotions (2001) is a visual model that helps us understand and categorise emotions. The wheel identifies eight primary emotions – joy, sadness, trust, disgust, fear, anger, surprise and anticipation – arranged to show their opposites and how they can combine to create more complex feelings. Each emotion also varies in intensity; for example, annoyance can escalate to anger, which in turn can intensify into rage.

In restorative supervision, Plutchik's Wheel can be a valuable tool for helping staff articulate and explore their emotional responses. It encourages deeper emotional awareness, supports regulation and fosters empathetic dialogue – especially when supervisees struggle to express what they're feeling or when emotions are layered and complex.

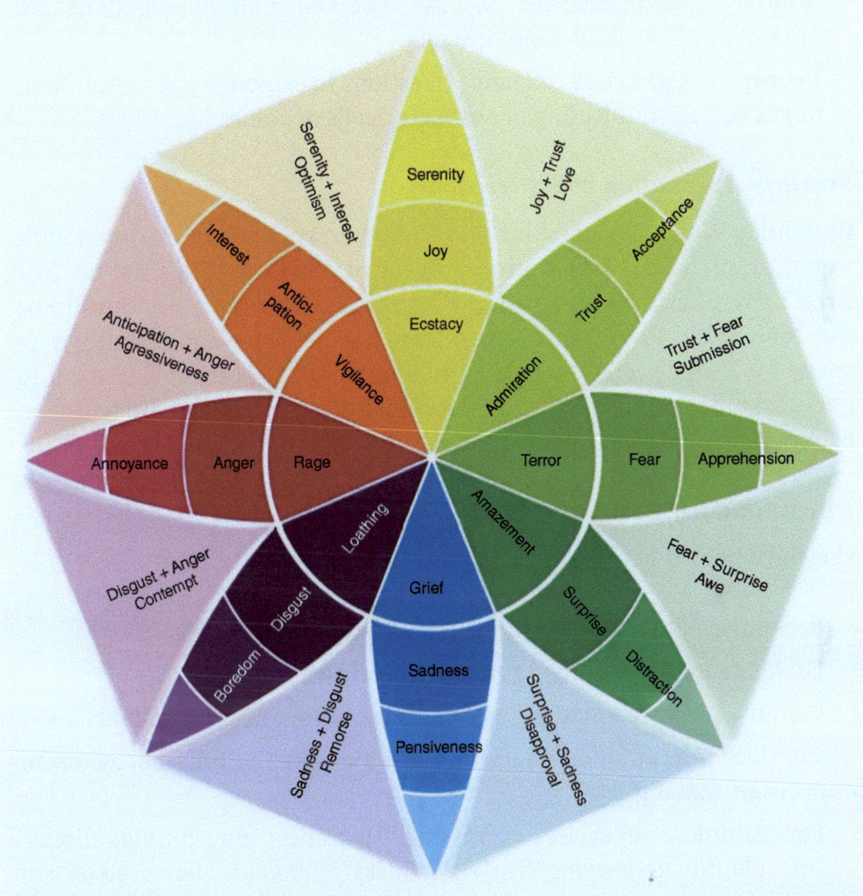

Dr Robert Plutchik's Wheel of Emotions

(continued)

(*continued*)

Instructions for Use

Introduce the Wheel: Share the visual model and explain the eight core emotions and their intensities.

Invite Reflection: Ask the supervisee to identify which emotion(s) they are experiencing in relation to a specific situation.

Explore Intensity: Encourage them to rate the strength of the emotion – mild, moderate or intense.

Identify Combinations: Discuss whether multiple emotions are present and how they might interact.

Prompt Insight: Use reflective questions to explore what the emotion might be communicating about their needs or values.

Practical Application in Supervision

Plutchik's Wheel is particularly useful when supervisees respond with vague or surface-level emotional descriptions (e.g. 'I'm fine' or 'just tired'). By offering a structured way to name and explore emotions, the tool helps PNAs and supervisors create a psychologically safe space for deeper reflection. It can be used at the start of a session to check in emotionally or during debriefs following challenging clinical experiences.

Discuss and Reframe

Use the wheel to help supervisees:

Recognise patterns in emotional responses.

Understand the underlying causes of their feelings.

Reframe negative emotions as signals for unmet needs or values.

Consider how emotional intensity may be affecting their behaviour or decision-making.

For example, a supervisee expressing 'frustration' may, through discussion, identify underlying 'fear' or 'sadness' related to a perceived lack of control or support.

Develop Action Plans

Once emotions are named and understood, guide the supervisee to:

Identify coping strategies or support systems that can help regulate intense emotions.

Set boundaries or make changes that address the root causes of emotional distress.

Plan follow-up actions, such as peer conversations, reflective journaling or well-being activities.

Developing a Growth Mindset

Overview of the Tool

A growth mindset, as defined by Carol Dweck (2006), is the belief that abilities and intelligence can be developed through effort, learning and persistence. In contrast, a fixed mindset assumes that talents are innate and unchangeable, often leading individuals to avoid challenges or give up easily. Within clinical supervision, fostering a growth mindset supports resilience, adaptability and professional development.

As PNAs and supervisees progress through their roles, they encounter new skills, responsibilities and emotional demands. Reflecting regularly on mindset – how one responds to feedback, mistakes and challenges – can help build intrinsic motivation and a culture of learning. Shifting mindset is not instantaneous; it requires emotional labour, self-awareness and intentional practice. Supervisors can use this tool to help staff reframe limiting beliefs and encourage growth-oriented thinking.

Instructions for Use

1. **Introduce the Concept:** Explain the difference between fixed and growth mindsets using simple examples.

2. **Use Reframing Statements:** Share common fixed mindset thoughts and their growth-oriented alternatives.

3. **Invite Reflection:** Ask the supervisee to consider how they typically respond to challenges, feedback and failure.

(continued)

(continued)

4. **Explore Motivation:** Discuss what drives their learning – external validation or internal growth?

5. **Encourage Self-awareness:** Use reflective prompts to deepen understanding of personal mindset patterns.

Practical Application in Supervision

This tool is especially useful when supervisees express self-doubt, fear of failure, or resistance to feedback. It can be used to:

- Support staff during transitions or new responsibilities.
- Reframe mistakes as learning opportunities.
- Encourage persistence and curiosity.
- Promote a team culture that values development over perfection.

Discuss and Reframe

Use the following reframing examples to guide discussion:

Fixed Mindset Thought	Reframed Growth Mindset Thought
'I'm not good at this'.	'I can improve with practice and effort'.
'I'll never get this right'.	'Mistakes help me learn and get better'.
'This is too hard'.	'This is challenging, and I can work through it'.
'I'm just not a natural at this'.	'I can develop my skills with persistence'.
'If I fail, it means I'm not capable'.	'Failure is an opportunity to grow and learn'.

Develop Action Plans

Support supervisees to:

- Identify one area where they'd like to shift from a fixed to a growth mindset.
- Set a small, achievable goal that requires effort and persistence.
- Practice reframing self-talk during challenges.
- Reflect on progress in future supervision sessions.
- Model growth mindset language and behaviours within their team.

The Coping Reservoir

Overview of the Tool

The coping reservoir (Dunn et al. 2008) is a metaphor for our overall well-being and psychological capacity to handle stress – a dynamic internal resource that holds the emotional, psychological and physical energy we draw upon to manage the demands of life and work. It's filled with the things that make us ourselves: our values, relationships, passions and sense of purpose. Positive inputs (like connection, mentorship, rest and achievement) replenish the reservoir, while negative inputs (like stress, isolation and moral distress) drain it. When the reservoir is balanced, we function well. But when reserves run low and are not replenished, we risk burnout, fatigue and disengagement. The goal is to maintain equilibrium by regularly topping up the reservoir with meaningful, restorative experiences.

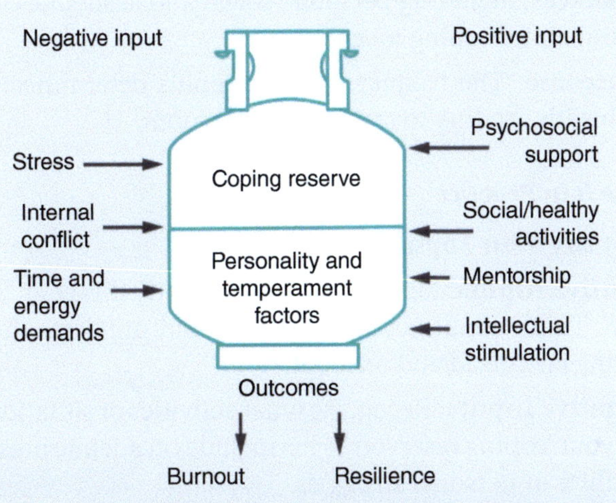

The Coping Reservoir. *Source:* Dunn et al. (2008) / with permission of Springer Nature

Using the Coping Reservoir in Clinical Supervision

To use the Coping Reservoir Model in practice, focus on identifying the positive and negative inputs that fill or drain the reservoir of your personal resources, which includes your personality, temperament and coping style. To fill the reservoir, practice adaptive coping by seeking support,

(continued)

(*continued*)

engaging in healthy activities like exercise and fostering self-awareness. To prevent draining, address maladaptive coping, such as social media overuse and avoiding self-care, which deplete your resources.

Understanding the Model

The Reservoir: This represents your psychological capacity to handle stress.

Inputs: Factors that either fill or drain the reservoir.

Positive Inputs (Filling): Activities and resources that replenish your well-being, such as strong relationships, mentorship, self-care and healthy activities (e.g. exercise and time outdoors).

Negative Inputs (Draining): Stressors and behaviours that deplete your resources, including personal, social and academic challenges, as well as unhelpful coping mechanisms.

The Outcome: The balance of these inputs determines your overall mental health, leading to resilience or burnout.

How to Use It in Practice

1. **Identify Your Inputs**:

   Positive Inputs: Reflect on what currently fills your 'coping reservoir'. Think about activities, people and mindsets that leave you feeling energized and resilient.

   Negative Inputs: Recognise what activities or situations are draining your 'coping reservoir'. This includes academic pressures, social conflicts or personal struggles.

2. **Monitor Your Reservoir's State:**

   Assess the balance – How full does your reservoir feel right now?

   Be aware of when you feel overwhelmed (reservoir is low) or when you have plenty of energy (reservoir is full).

   Use a scale (e.g. 1–10) or visual imagery to help them express this.

3. **Implement Strategies to Fill the Reservoir:**

   Discuss what activities, connection or relationships help to fill the reservoir.

Seek Support: Connect with family, friends, mentors or support groups.

Prioritise Self-Care: Schedule time for exercise, hobbies, rest and activities that bring you joy.

Practice Mindfulness and Reflection: Journaling, spending time in nature or engaging in other reflective practices can help build your resources.

Try to identify small realistic steps, e.g. scheduling breaks, seeking peer support and engaging in hobbies.

4. **Develop Strategies to Prevent Draining:**

   Limit Unhelpful Coping: Reduce or avoid behaviours that drain your energy, such as excessive social media use or news consumption.

   Develop Self-Awareness: Understand your personal triggers and how they affect your stress levels.

   Cultivate a Positive Outlook: Try to reframe challenges and look forward to the future.

5. **Create an Action Plan**

   Agree on one or two actions to support replenishment before the next supervision.

   Revisit the reservoir metaphor regularly to track changes and support resilience.

(Yerkes-Dodson Law)

Overview of the Tool

The Stress Curve, based on Yerkes-Dodson Law (1908), illustrates the relationship between pressure and performance. It shows that while moderate stress can enhance focus and productivity, excessive or prolonged stress impairs cognitive function, decision-making and emotional regulation – ultimately leading to burnout. The curve is typically divided into three zones: low pressure (under-stimulation), optimal pressure (peak performance) and high pressure (overload and decline).

(continued)

(*continued*)

In clinical practice, stress often builds gradually and unnoticed. Many professionals adapt to rising demands, normalising chronic stress and internalising it as personal failure. This mindset can mask the early signs of burnout, which carries emotional, physical and professional risks – including increased likelihood of clinical errors. PNAs and supervisors can use the stress curve to help staff visualise their current stress levels, reflect on their coping strategies and intervene before crisis point.

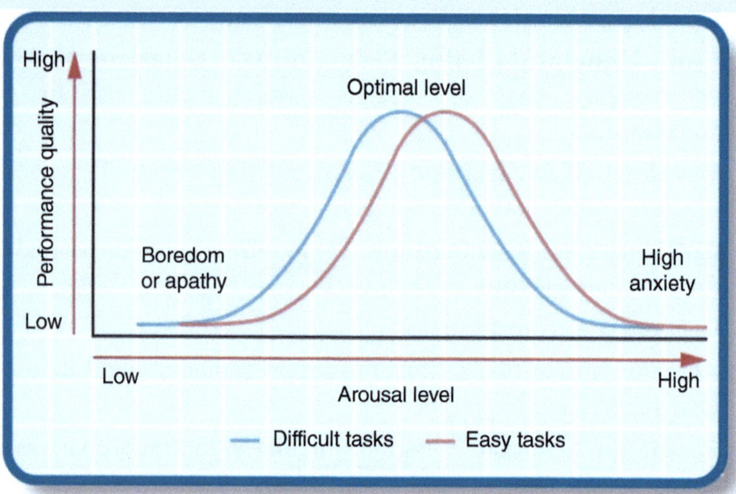

Source: Adapted from Yerkes and Dodson (1908)

Instructions for Use

1. **Introduce the Curve**: Share the Yerkes-Dodson diagram and explain the three zones of pressure.

2. **Invite Self-Assessment:** Ask the supervisee to identify where they currently sit on the curve.

3. **Explore Contributing Factors:** Discuss what's driving their current stress level – both internal and external.

4. **Identify Early Warning Signs**: Help them recognise physical, emotional, and behavioural indicators of rising stress.

5. **Prompt Reflection**: Use guided questions to explore how they typically respond to increasing pressure.

Practical Application in Supervision

The stress curve is particularly effective in helping supervisees visualise the tipping point between productive stress and harmful overload. It can be used during supervision to:

- Debrief after high-pressure situations.
- Explore patterns of overwork or perfectionism.
- Normalise conversations about stress and well-being.
- Support early intervention and recovery planning.

Discuss and Reframe

Use the curve to help supervisees:

- Reframe stress as a physiological and psychological response – not a personal weakness.
- Recognise that performance decline under stress is predictable and reversible.
- Reflect on protective factors they may be neglecting (e.g. rest, connection and hobbies).
- Consider how their current coping strategies may be helping or hindering recovery.

For example, a supervisee who responds to stress by working longer hours may realise they're sacrificing restorative activities that would actually improve performance and well-being.

Develop Action Plans

Guide the supervisee to:

- Identify one or two protective factors they can reintroduce (e.g. regular breaks and peer support).
- Set realistic boundaries around work and rest.

(continued)

(*continued*)

- Plan a check-in or follow-up supervision to monitor stress levels.
- Consider team-level conversations to promote a culture of well-being and early support.

Finding the Joy in Your Work

Overview of the Tool

Joy in work (Daisley 2019) is not a luxury – it is a foundational element of sustainable, compassionate healthcare practice. For PNAs, rediscovering joy can restore emotional balance, build resilience and foster a culture of well-being. Joy is often found in moments of connection, purpose, and recognition, and when nurses feel valued and engaged in meaningful work, they are more likely to experience fulfilment and less likely to burn out.

The Institute for Healthcare Improvement (IHI) frames joy in work as a system-level concern, not just an individual one. Their approach encourages leaders and teams to ask, 'What matters to you?' – a question PNAs can use to open reflective conversations and uncover what brings meaning and satisfaction to their colleagues (Perlo et al. 2017). Rather than waiting for joy to appear, PNAs can help create the conditions for it: psychological safety, peer support, autonomy and opportunities for reflection. These elements not only improve morale but also enhance patient care and team cohesion.

Instructions for Use

1. **Introduce the Concept**: Explain that joy in work is essential for well-being and performance, not a bonus.
2. **Use the '*What Matters to You?*' Question**: Invite supervisees to reflect on what brings meaning and satisfaction to their role.
3. **Explore Joyful Moments:** Ask them to recall recent experiences of joy or fulfilment at work.
4. **Identify Barriers and Enablers**: Discuss what helps or hinders joy in their current environment.
5. **Encourage Reflection**: Use prompts to deepen understanding of personal and professional values.

Practical Application in Supervision

This tool is especially effective when supervisees feel disconnected, demotivated or overwhelmed. It can be used to:

- Reconnect staff with the meaningful aspects of their role.
- Promote well-being and emotional recovery.
- Support team culture by encouraging shared values and appreciation.
- Identify small, actionable changes that enhance joy and engagement.

Discuss and Reframe

Use reflective dialogue to help supervisees:

- Recognise that joy is a legitimate and necessary part of professional life.
- Reframe joy as a protective factor against burnout.
- Explore how small moments of connection or purpose can have a big impact.
- Consider how they can contribute to a joyful team culture.

For example, a supervisee who feels undervalued may, through reflection, identify that peer recognition or patient feedback helps restore their sense of purpose.

Super Helper Syndrome

Overview of the Tool

Super Helper Syndrome (Baker and Vincent 2022) refers to a pattern where individuals overextend themselves in their desire to help others – often at the expense of their own well-being. This is particularly relevant in the NHS and caring professions, where many professionals, including PNAs, are drawn to roles that involve emotional and expert support. While helping is a core value, unchecked helping behaviours can lead to compassion fatigue, burnout and a diminished capacity to care effectively.

The model identifies four types of help:

- Resource-based (providing tools, labour and materials)
- Informational (sharing knowledge)

(continued)

(*continued*)

- Expert help (clinical or professional expertise)
- Supportive help (emotional encouragement)

PNAs often gravitate toward expert and supportive help, making them especially vulnerable. Super helpers may hold irrational beliefs about what it means to be a 'good person' or 'good nurse', struggling to say no or set boundaries. Baker and Vincent encourage professionals to challenge these beliefs and recognise their own bandwidth or available emotional and cognitive capacity. Recognising capacity and setting boundaries is essential in sustaining compassionate practice and avoiding overwhelm.

Instructions for Use

Introduce the Concept: Explain Super Helper Syndrome and the four types of help.

- **Explore Beliefs**: Invite supervisees to reflect on their internal rules or expectations around helping.
- **Assess Bandwidth**: Use metaphors like dashboard lights or stereo volume to help them visualise their current capacity.
- **Identify Patterns**: Discuss which types of help they offer most often and how it affects their energy.
- **Encourage Boundary Setting**: Support supervisees in identifying where they need to say no or step back.

Practical Application in Supervision

This tool is particularly useful when supervisees show signs of overcommitment, emotional exhaustion or difficulty delegating. It can be used to:

- Normalise conversations about limits and boundaries.
- Explore the emotional cost of constant helping.
- Support supervisees in recognising their own needs.
- Encourage sustainable helping behaviours that protect well-being.

Discuss and Reframe

Use reflective dialogue to help supervisees:

- Challenge unrealistic beliefs about being 'good' or 'indispensable'.
- Reframe boundary setting as a professional strength, not a failure.

- Recognise that saying no can be an act of care – for themselves and others.
- Explore how different types of help impact their energy and effectiveness.

For example, a supervisee who always offers emotional support may realise they're neglecting their own emotional needs and need to rebalance their helping style.

Develop Action Plans

Support supervisees to:

- Identify one area where they can set or reinforce a boundary.
- Reflect on which types of help they can offer sustainably.
- Practice saying no or delegating in a supportive environment.
- Monitor their bandwidth and adjust commitments accordingly.
- Plan follow-up supervision to reflect on progress and well-being.

Building Your Network and Support

The role of the PNA is not to solve every problem, nor to provide coaching or counselling. Instead, effective PNAs draw on the strength of a network or community of practice, which serves as a repository of shared learning as well as a source of tools, resources and support. Many of these resources can be signposted during supervision sessions to enhance impact. As the role becomes more established across healthcare settings, lead PNAs and local support networks are emerging. In addition, national resources are available through National NHS Collaboration Platforms, which are particularly valuable for those working in more isolated practice. Below is a list of suggested resources to consider as part of your own PNA toolbox or network. This list is not exhaustive and will vary by region, so a good starting point is to explore your employing organisation's well-being offer and what is available locally. For newly qualified PNAs, making early connections with key individuals or teams, such as Freedom to Speak Up Guardians, can also provide vital support and guidance.

Tool Box

NHS Civility & Respect Framework

NHS Civility & Respect Toolkit

NHS Core Values & Organisational Values

NHS People Plan 2021

NHS People Promise

NHS Health & Wellbeing Implementation Guide

NHSE Employers Retention Toolkit NHS Retention Hub

NHS Leadership Academy: Team Resilience Hub

NHSE PNA

NHSE PNA Checklists

NHS Workplace Compassion Support Pack 2020 The Courage of
Compassion, The Kings Fund

NHSE Freedom to Speak Up 2022

Lees-Deutsch Toolkit Leadership Development Offer

RCN Standards for Education & Training 2023

ELfH PNA Portal

FONS: Resilience Based Clinical Supervision

Mental Health First Aid

Shiny Mind

NHS Headspace

Schwartz Rounds

Network

Lead PNA – PNA network

Freedom to Speak up

PALS

NHS Collaboration Platforms

Mental Health First Aider

Organisational Development

Continuing Education Team

Occupational Health

Wellbeing Lead

REFERENCES

Applewhite, C. and Logan, J. (2022). *Adult Critical Care Services: Professional Nurse Advocate Toolkit*. Manchester University `https:// www.cc3n.org.uk/uploads/9/8/4/2/98425184/pna_restorative_ clinical_supervision_tool_kit.pdf`.

Baker, J. and Vincent, R. (2022). *The Super-Helper Syndrome: A Survival Guide for Compassionate People*. Flint.

Beckwith, M. (2022). *A Pilot Evaluation of the Professional Nurse Advocate (PNA) Programme in Adult Critical Care: A mixed-methods approach*. University of Leeds.

Beinart, H. and Clohessy, S. (2016). Clinical supervision. In: *Case Formulation in Cognitive Behaviour Therapy: The Treatment of Challenging and Complex Cases*, 2e (ed. N. Tarrier and J. Johnson), 352–369. Routledge/Taylor & Francis Group.

Brockman, R., Ciarrochi, J., Parker, P., and Kashdan, T. (2016). Emotion regulation strategies in daily life: mindfulness, cognitive reappraisal and emotion suppression. *Cognitive Behaviour Therapy* 46 (2): 91–113. `https:// doi.org/10.1080/16506073.2016.1218926`.

Butterworth, T. (2022). What is clinical supervision and how can it be delivered in practice? *Nursing Times* 118 (2): 20–22.

Butterworth, T. and Fougier, J. (1992). Clinical supervision as an emerging idea in nursing. Springer Science and Business Media. `http://ndl. ethernet.edu.et/bitstream/123456789/1379/1/Tony% 20Butterworth.pdf#page=11` (accessed on 03 September 2025).

Cannon, W.B. (1929). Organization for physiological homeostasis. *Physiological Reviews* 9: 399–431. `https://doi.org/10.1152/physrev.1929. 9.3.399`.

Carragher, L. and Gormley, K. (2017). Leadership and emotional intelligence in nursing. *Nursing Management* 24 (8): 32–37.

Copp, G. (1988). The reality behind stress. *Nursing Times* 84 (45): 50–53.

Covey, S. (1989). *The 7 Habits of Highly Effective People: Powerful Lessons in Personal Change*. New York: Simon & Schuster.

Daisley, B. (2019). *The Joy of Work*. UK: Penguin Random House.

Doucette, P.A. (2004). Walk and talk: an intervention for behaviourally challenged youths. *Adolescence* 39 (154): 373.

Dunn, L.B., Iglewicz, A., and Moutier, C. (2008). A conceptual model of medical student well-being: promoting resilience and preventing burnout. *Academic Psychiatry* 32 (1): 44–53. https://doi.org/10.1176/appi.ap.32.1.44.

Dweck, C. (2006). *Mindset: The New Psychology of Success*. New York: Balantine Books.

Ekman, P. (1999). Basic emotions. In: *Handbook of Cognition and Emotion* (ed. T. Dalgleish and M.J. Power), 45–60. John Wiley & Sons Ltd. https://doi.org/10.1002/0470013494.ch3.

Figley, C.R. (1995). *Compassion Fatigue: Coping with Secondary Traumatic Stress Disorder in Those Who Treat the Traumatized*. Brunner/Mazel.

Fox, E. (2008). *Emotion Science Cognitive and Neuroscientific Approaches to Understanding Human Emotions*. Palgrave Macmillan. ISBN: 978-0-230-00517-4.

Gibbs, G. (1988). *Learning by Doing: A Guide to Teaching and Learning Methods*. Oxford: Further Education Unit, Oxford Polytechnic.

Goleman, D. (2000). *Emotional Intelligence: Why It Can Matter More Than IQ*. London: Bloomsbury Publishing.

Griffiths, K. (2022). Using restorative supervision to help nurses during the Covid-19 pandemic. *Nursing Times* 118: 3.

Hill, J. (1989). Supervision in the caring professions: a literature review. *Community Psychiatric Nursing Journal* 9 (5): 9–15.

Hochschild, A.R. (1983). *The Managed Heart: Commercialization of Human Feeling*. Berkeley, CA: University of California Press.

Houlihan, G., Keane, V., and Thomas, A. (2022). The implementation of restorative clinical supervision to support every voice being heard. *Archives of Disease in Childhood* 108 (1): https://doi.org/10.1136/archdischild-2023-gosh.8.

Johns, C. (1995). Framing Learning through Reflection within Carper's Fundamental Ways of Knowing in Nursing. 22 (2): 226–234. https://doi.org/10.1046/j.1365-2648.1995.22020226.x.

Johnson, J., Corker, C., and O'Connor, D. (2020). Burnout in psychological therapists: A cross-sectional study investigating the role of supervisory relationship quality. *Clinical Psychologist* 24: 223–235. https://doi.org/10.1111/cp.12206.

Kahneman, D. (2011). Part 1: Chapter 1 The Characters of the story. In: *Thinking, Fast and Slow* (ed. A. Lane), 18–21. England: Macmillan.

King's Fund (2025). NHS staff wellbeing and burnout. https://www.kingsfund.org.uk/ (accessed 03 September 2025).

Lainidi, O., Johnson, J., Griffin, B. et al. (2025). Associations between burnout, employee silence and voice: a systematic review and meta-analysis. *Psychology & Health* https://doi.org/10.1080/08870446.2025.2509074.

Lees-Deutsch, L., Palmer, S., Adegboye, A. et al. (2023) National Evaluation Report of the Professional Nurse Advocate Programme: Mixed Methods Study. https://pureportal.coventry.ac.uk/files/70132294/REPORT_Final_June_2023.pdf (accessed on 03 September 2025).

Lees-Deutsch, L., Palmer, S., Rodrigues Amorim Adegboye, A. et al. (2025). Professional nurse advocates and restorative clinical supervision: national survey of programme implementation and impact. *BMC Nursing* https://doi.org/10.1186/s12912-025-03415-z.

Liedgren, J., Pieter, M.A., and Gaggioli, A. (2023). Liminal design: a conceptual framework and three-step approach for developing technology that delivers transcendence and deeper experiences. *Frontiers in Psychology* 14: 1043170. https://doi.org/10.3389/fpsyg.2023.10.3170.

Lockwood, T. (2024). Reflective leadership in nursing supervision. *Nurse Leader Journal* 12 (1): 15–22.

MacLean, P.D. (1990). *The Triune Brain in Evolution: Role in Paleo Cerebral Functions*. New York: Plenum Press bbm:978-1-4615-4271-1/1.pdf (springer.com).

Martin, R. and Milne, D. (2018). Authentic leadership in clinical supervision. *Clinical Supervision Review* 26 (3): 120–130.

Masamha, R., Alfred, A., Harris, R. et al. (2022). 'Barriers to overcoming the barriers': a scoping review exploring 30 years of clinical supervision literature. *The Journal of Advanced Nursing* https://doi.org/10.1111/jan.15283.

McKinney, B.L. (2011) Therapists perceptions of walk and talk therapy: A grounded study. Dissertations & Thesis. University of New Orleans Theses and Dissertations.

NHS Digital (2024). NHS Sickness Absence Statistics. https://digital.nhs.uk/data-and-information/publications/statistical/nhs-sickness-absence-rates/december-2024#chapter-index (accessed 03 September 2025).

NHS England (2020). The NHS people plan: our people promise. https://www.england.nhs.uk/our-nhs-people/online-version/lfaop/our-nhs-people-promise/ (accessed on 03 September 2025).

NHS England (2021). A-EQUIP a model of clinical midwifery supervision. `https://www.england.nhs.uk/wp-content/uploads/2017/04/a-equip-midwifery-supervision-model.pdf` (accessed on 03 September 2025).

NHS England (2022). Professional nurse advocate. `https://www.england.nhs.uk/nursingmidwifery/delivering-the-nhs-ltp/professional-nurse-advocate/` (accessed 03 September 2025).

Nuffield Trust (2025). NHS staff survey: positive improvements but worrying trends on staff wellbeing remain. `https://www.nuffieldtrust.org.uk/news-item/nhs-staff-survey-positive-improvements-but-worrying-trends-on-staff-wellbeing-remain` (accessed 03 September 2025).

Nursing and Midwifery Council (2018). The Code: Professional standards of practice and behaviour for nurses, midwives and nursing associates. `https://www.nmc.org.uk/globalassets/sitedocuments/nmc-publications/nmc-code.pdf` (accessed on 03 September 2025).

Perlo, J., Balik, B., Swensen, S. et al. (2017). IHI framework for improving joy in work. Institute for Healthcare Improvement. `https://www.ihi.org/library/white-papers/ihi-framework-improving-joy-work#:~:text=The%20first%20step%20to%20improving,leaders%20prepare%20for%20these%20conversations.` (accessed 03 September 2025).

Pettit, A. and Stephen, R. (2015). *Supporting Health Visitors and Fostering Resilience Literature Review*. London: Institute of Health Visiting `https://healthvisitors.wordpress.com/wp-content/uploads/2015/03/ihv_literature-review_v9.pdf`.

Plutchik, R. (2001). The Nature of Emotions: Human emotions have deep evolutionary roots, a fact that may explain their complexity and provide tools for clinical practice. *American Scientist* 89 (4): 344–350. `http://www.jstor.org/stable/27857503`.

Revell, S. (2017). Walk and talk therapy: potential client perceptions. *Contemporary Research Topics* 24.

Rolfe, G., Freshwater, D., and Jasper, M. (2001). *Critical Reflection for Nursing and the Helping Professions: A User's Guide*. Palgrave Macmillan.

Rouse, S. (2019). The role of the PMA and barriers to the successful implementation of restorative clinical supervision. *British Journal of MIdwifery*. 27: 6.

Royal College of Nursing (2022). Position statement on clinical supervision. https://www.rcn.org.uk/About-us/Our-Influencing-work/Position-statements/rcn-position-on-clinical-supervision (accessed 03 September 2025).

Royal College of Nursing (2024). *Stress and Sickness Absence in the Nursing Workforce: Annual Workforce Report 2024.* London: RCN https://www.rcn.org.uk/news-and-events/Press-Releases/nhs-sickness-data-shows-average-nurse-took-entire-week-off-sick-last-year-stress-apr24.

Scanlon, M. and Hart, T. (2024). Wellbeing of self and others: key considerations in restorative supervision. *Nursing Times* 120 (5).

Talbot, S.M. (2007). *The Cortisol Connection: Why Stress Makes You Fat and Ruins Your Health – and What You Can Do About It.* Berkeley, CA: Hunter House.

Valentino, A.L., LeBlanc, L.A., Sellers, T.P. et al. (2016). The benefits of group supervision and a recommendation for implementation. *Behaviour Analysis in Practice* 9 (4): 320–328.

van den Agnes, B. and Beute, F. (2021). Walk it off! The effectiveness of walk and talk coaching in nature for individuals with burnout and stress-related complaints. *Clinical Therapeutics* 4: 473. https://doi.org/10.1016/j.jenvp.2021.101641.

Wallbank, S. (2010). Effectiveness of individual clinical supervision for midwives and doctors in stress reduction: findings from a pilot study. *Evidence Based Midwifery* 8: 65–70.

Wallbank, S. and Hatton, S. (2011). Evaluation of clinical supervision using the restorative model. *Clinical Psychology Forum* 22 (3): 20–26.

Wallbank, S. and Robertson, N. (2008). Midwife and nurse responses to miscarriage, stillbirth and neonatal death: a critical review of qualitative research. *Evidence Based Midwifery* 6 (3): 100–106.

Wallbank, S. and Woods, G. (2012). A healthier health visiting workforce. Findings from the Restorative Supervision Programme. *Community Practitioner* 85 (11): 20–23. https://www.researchgate.net/publication/233937804_A_healthier_health_visiting_workforce_Findings_from_the_restorative_supervision_programme.

West, M. and Chowla, R. (2017). *Compassionate Leadership: Sustaining Wisdom, Humanity and Presence in Health and Care.* The King's Fund.

West, M., Bailey, S., and Williams, E. (2020). *The Courage of Compassion: Supporting Nurse and Midwives to Deliver High-Quality Care.* The King's Fund.

Yerkes, R.M. and Dodson, J.D. (1908). The relation of strength of stimulus to rapidity of habit-formation. *Journal of Comparative Neurology and Psychology* 18 (5): 459–482.

CHAPTER 6

A Reflective Journey Through Quality Improvement for PNAs

Martin Hogan

The Improvement Coalition CIC, London, UK

INTRODUCTION: QUALITY IMPROVEMENT FOR PROFESSIONAL NURSE ADVOCATES

Working within today's fast-paced and often stressful health and care systems, professional nurse advocates (PNAs) play a vital role in championing the needs of healthcare staff while ensuring the care needs of individuals and communities are met. They do this by advocating for patients, supporting staff, and driving wider system improvements. The work of a PNA closely aligns with quality improvement (QI) principles, ensuring that services remain safe, effective, equitable and continuously improving.

Despite this alignment, many PNAs here may not view themselves as quality improvers or agents of change – even though their daily efforts often identify gaps in care, enhance outcomes and strengthen both patient and staff experiences. This may be partly due to the early focus of the PNA role to provide restorative clinical supervision (RCS), rather than on system-level improvement.

QI should also be seen as a restorative skill set – an essential tool for supporting those we care for. It is recognised as one of the four key pillars of PNA practice and is fundamental to developing confidence, improving safety and fostering a culture of continuous learning. In the current climate of

---

This chapter is written in a conversational and informal style.

political and organisational change, these skills are more important than ever. The ability to think critically, reflect, measure, evaluate and implement improvements across systems is crucial to the success of our workforce, the safety of our patients and the sustainability of our services.

In health care, QI is an established methodology that systematically enhances outcomes for patients, staff and organisations. As defined by Southern New Hampshire University (2024), 'QI tools can significantly improve healthcare delivery by saving time, enhancing timeliness, reducing costs and minimising errors'. At a time of financial constraint, growing service demand and workforce pressures, QI offers powerful opportunities to improve both quality and productivity.

Whether you are new to QI or already applying its principles, this chapter will provide practical tools and guidance to help you become a more confident PNA and drive meaningful, sustainable change. Many PNAs express uncertainty around QI, asking questions such as: 'Am I doing it correctly?', 'What if I get it wrong?' or 'Is this just another thing to add to my workload?' My response is simple – learning new skills always involves making mistakes. My experience suggests that by removing the words *I can't* from your vocabulary; they reflect a fixed mindset. Instead, replace them with *I don't know how... yet*. Growth begins with curiosity and persistence – and QI is all about growth.

This chapter will take you on a journey exploring how PNAs can use QI methodologies to strengthen their practice, improve patient outcomes and enhance experiences across the system. It will introduce key QI concepts and tools, demonstrating how they can help identify problems, generate solutions and influence change at every level. My personal reflections, real-life examples and practical strategies will illustrate how PNAs can confidently apply QI principles in everyday practice and lead meaningful improvements.

By the end of this chapter, readers will:

- Understand the connection between PNAs and QI.
- Gain insights into core QI principles.
- Know how to run a QI project.
- Learn practical techniques for identifying, measuring and addressing areas for improvement.
- Explore strategies for influencing change in ever-evolving environments.

LEARNING THE LANGUAGE

In the world of QI, there are lots of new key words and phrases used to describe QI methodologies, which are described here:

The Purists and the Pirate

This was conceived by me, as I kept being told off by proper data capturers. They kept saying, 'this is not pure data Martin!' to which I replied, 'I'm not a purist, I'm a pirate, and ever after I have sailed the seas of QI as proud pirate!'

The purist's mentality relates to people who must have all the details the exact way it was relayed to them and follow QI rules to the letter. The pirate mentality relates to people who have been given an idea and follow a create, self taught pathway to achieve the same results. They creatively get from A to B, but they truly get from A to B their way, and different approaches to QI will work. Our difference is our collective PNA superpower.

Stakeholders

This phrase can be heard extensively in the world of executive and continuous improvement. In QI, a stakeholder is properly defined as any individual, group or organisation that can affect or is affected by a QI initiative. Stakeholders play a crucial role in shaping the project's direction, ensuring relevance to practice, supporting implementation and helping to sustain changes over time. Their involvement is essential for identifying problems, co-designing solutions, facilitating adoption and ensuring that improvement efforts are aligned with the needs and expectations of those impacted.

You will often also hear three words used to describe the type of involvement with projects.

These are co-production, co-design and co-convene.

This is helpful to know as you can understand who has been involved in shaping the project and to what extent.

Co-production: With stakeholders means that stakeholders have been engaged with project ideas from the beginning and throughout various milestones of the project.

Having ideas and updates presented to them with the stakeholder's opinions being listened to.

As healthcare professionals, we co-produce care plans with patients and their loved ones all the time. We also lead family meeting with members of the multidisciplinary team to co-produce treatment plans, complex discharges and end-of-life care decisions. The phrase commonly said in practice is 'no conversation about me, without me'. I think we should all remember this is a golden rule when undertaking QI projects. If we are undertaking QI that impacts patients, why would we not involve them as key stakeholders. True QI should always have patients as stakeholders or project partners as this is proved to ensure that the project is more relevant, sustainable and equitable for the better of the communities in which we serve (BMJ 2023).

Co-design: Refers to stakeholders' designing the project with you as the project lead, influencing the project at all of its milestones. For example, children who had been patients were asked to co-design the next hospital with the architects from the beginning of the project and kept involved throughout major milestones of the project, which really helped the success of the building and in reducing anxiety around hospital admissions, as the new hospital felt like a playroom due to the children patient stakeholder's involvement.

Co-convening: Refers to stakeholders who share responsibility for organising and running a project.

At the end of all QI projects, I think it's important to share learning with stakeholders, but also the wider audience. Whether the project was a success or not. Learning from failure is such a valuable experience as PNAs. For example, this can be reflected upon and applied to all functions of our practice learning – from an RCS session that didn't go so well or a QI project that you couldn't get off the ground. Understanding the cause of failed QI work and impact allows us to continuously improve, and if we are continuously improving, we are continuously growing.

It can be seen as best practice to have patients and people with lived experienced of service use, involved as key stakeholders in all QI projects. When this is possible (as not all QI does involve patients), the likelihood of success, sustainability, reach and equity within your project is increased by 100% (BMJ 2023).

The PDSA Cycle

Plan, do, study, act is known as PDSA, which was invented by Langley et al. (2009) as an iterative cycle for testing change. It very simply advises you to:

    a. Plan what you are going to do.
    b. Do what you want to change.
    c. Study what you are changing.
    d. Then act upon it.

This is a cyclical process where users of a PDSA cycle can repeat the work using different measures to improve the outcomes they set out to achieve through the QI work. There can be a danger of not knowing when to draw the work to a reasonable conclusion.

An easier place to start, but one that may be less familiar to readers, is this simple six-step approach I have developed and used to avoid over complicating matters:

1. What do you want to change?
2. Why do you want to change it?
3. How are you going to change it?
4. Who is going to help you change it?
5. How will you know when your change has been successful?
6. And does it need to be successful?

Each step may require supportive approaches, which are also described here:

1. **What do you want to change?**
   Think about what it is you want to change.

   Is this change a priority and why is it being prioritised? Is it realistic? It is important that when we are undertaking QI or supporting others to do so. To achieve change requires an understanding of the contextual factors and that we are aware of these in order to know what change we tackle first. So, we need to think SMART!

What Is a SMART Aim?

A **SMART aim** is a clearly defined goal for your improvement project that is:

- **Specific**: Focused and unambiguous.
- **Measurable**: Quantifiable, with clear criteria for success.
- **Achievable:** Realistic given the time and resources available.
- **Relevant:** Aligned with broader priorities and the problem you're trying to solve.
- **Time-bound:** Includes a clear deadline or timeframe.

(continued)

(*continued*)

SMART aims help teams stay focused, measure progress and evaluate success. A well-written SMART aim typically includes what you're trying to improve, by how much, for whom and by when.

Example: 'Reduce the number of patients missing their asthma check-up appointments at Clinic A by 30% by 31 December 2025'.

Before undertaking any project, write down your project idea using the SMART aim.

What you want to change will be invaluable to the project.

This methodology is your new best critical friend. We all need critical friends in QI.

Let's SMART critique!

- Yes, it is specific.
- yes, it is measurable.
- yes, it is achievable.
- Yes, it is relevant.
- Yes, it is timely.

As we have more yes responses than no this is SMART, so we can proceed on to the next step.

Having this ability to critique elements of QI as they build can be applied to RCS and career conversations (CC) as well. It can be used in all facets of leadership, think applying for a job or a course.

2. **Why do you want to change it?**

   Here we are trying to understand the cause and the effect of the problem.

   What is causing the problem, and what is affecting the problem?

   Understanding our why is critical when undertaking QI, as this allows for a firmer understanding of the complexities that may be encountered.

   QI methodology that is useful for this is 'the five whys'. Sakichi Toyoda, former founder of Toyota industries, invented this concept back in the early 20th century (Serrat 2009). This tool asks that you state the problem and then ask your why five times to get to the root cause of the problem. Do explain to people first what you are doing when using this, however, as why is often felt to be a critical question and might be received differently than intended. Why is often associated as passive aggressive or me as a 'stroppy teenager' talking back to my mum. Within the QI world, however, why is often the best question.

For example, our problem is the number of patients missing their asthma check-up appointments at the clinic. If we apply the five-whys approach, we can help better understand the cause and effect.

People are not attending asthma check-ups.

- Why? Because we don't run clinics at a time that suits most people who are at work.
- Why? Because our way of working only currently allows clinics to be Monday to Friday 9–5 p.m.
- Why? Because then staff would have to be paid unsocial hours, and there isn't a budget for that.
- Why? Because within our service we are only allowed to spend money if the service generates income.
- Why? Because that's what my boss says.
- Why? Because that's what her boss says.
- I have taken artistic license here to show you an example. However, in real life often the cause and effect mean we are working in systems strangled by budgets. Using the five whys, we can now get to the cause and effect, which helps us approach our quality improvement from a different angle or makes us re-evaluate if we even want to go near a problem with QI. There would be a cost to paying clinic staff unsocial pay. However, patients not attending clinic appointments costs the NHS well over 200 million pounds. By re-imaging the problem through a QI lens, we could be more efficient, provide safer and more equitable services to the communities we serve and be cost-effective.

3. **How are you going to change it?**
Having a plan for any project is invaluable, and I would advise an essential.

It does have to be neat and tidy – but do have a plan; life is complicated enough to try and remember everything.

For QI projects, tools, such as a Driver diagram (Institute for Healthcare 1990), are used to map the project and provide direction.

A Driver diagram for a PNA should start with the change ideas using a SMART aim. The purpose of the diagram is to support you through 'driving' a process for your change ideas. It also helps to make your process transparent for others to see and understand. In the process, there will be primary and secondary drivers of how and what you will need to have in place for your project to work (notice here I said work and not successful).

Controversial moment is that you start from the left to right.

I have given examples of how a QI project can be started and driven, but this links to the whole role of being a PNA and relies upon ideas being generated from RCS.

An example of how PNAs can transition from delivering RCS, identifying issues and translating into QI is offered through utilising the concepts of the snakes and ladders model, I invented. A National PNA Toolkit (Lees-Deutsch et al. 2025), developed as part of the evaluation of QI work within the PNA role, may also be very useful to guide the development of QI work in practice areas; this has several practical tools that align with some of the ideas presented here.

Much like a popular board game, I grew up so fondly playing the snakes and ladders game. This was a game where you had to get from the start to finish on a board. You rolled a dice, and each player got a go to roll with the aim to get your piece to the finish first. If you landed on a ladder, you could move further forward on the board. If you sadly landed on a snake, you had to go back on the board. Meaning, it made it harder for you to win. I always landed on a snake and sadly have never won a round of snakes and ladders.

However, the adult me drew familiarity with this board game and when delivering RCS as a professional advocate, I think to myself how do I move this RCS into a QI project? Eureka, I yelped. It reminded me of a game of snakes and ladders.

If in RCS, subject matter is discussed that you feel could be a QI project, you have landed on a ladder, which means you can take QI forward following RCS. Example of this would be that the supervisee has mentioned how bad their local induction was with their team. You could then ask them to put their change ideas down on paper. Once they have done that, then ask them how they are going to make those changes happen and so on and so on until you have your S.M.A.R.T. aim for a QI project.

In the formative section of RCS, you can use probing questions to check if a QI project can grow from what you have heard.

If, however, subject matter isn't appropriate to take a QI project forward, you have landed on a snake. Subject matters are best advised not to be made into QI projects from my experience having learnt the hard way.

1. Very simply ask those you supervise to write down their change ideas on a poster.

2. Then ask them if they see themes of change ideas and get them to group the change ideas into themes.
3. Then ask the supervisee how/what they will need to make that change happen.

These become secondary and primary drivers. As you can imagine, this process is very restorative, e.g. having visuals of your change ideas or problems gives people space to reflect. You as the professional advocate have utilised both RCS and QI methodology.

So, now QI will be taken forward.

Remember, not everything needs to be a QI project. Some things are best 'Just do the project, which might be a service improvement, audit or small-scale work not requiring the many tools used in QI'. Nevertheless, QI methodology can still be used as a tool to explore issues raised in RCS, such as the stinky fish model (<u>Hyper Island</u>).

This is a user-friendly and explorative model to better understand people's (staff and patient) issues. The image is you have brought fish in for lunch. You forget to eat your lunch that day and you leave it in the fridge. Some time passes and you have still forgotten your lunch is in the fridge. Your colleagues start complaining about the smell being stinky. You must take it out and throw it away. The longer you leave fish, the more smellier it becomes. The longer you ignore a problem, the bigger it gets. The stinky fish model asks four simple questions:

1. What are your uncertainties?
2. What is making you feel worried?
3. What are your past issues with this that you can't get over?
4. What are you thinking, but not saying?

This tool allows deeper reflection within RCS, CC or QI.

1. For example, you attend an RCS session with me. We spend an hour journeying through the A-equip model. Starting with our psychological safety contracting, boundary setting and agreeing our frequency and duration. Then it's over to you to discuss your agenda item (subject you wish to discuss in RCS). This is the restorative section of RCS. You mention in this section that you have a lot of stress at work at the minute and your boss is breathing down your neck to make improvements. Your asthma clinic has poor attendance, and Clinical Quality Commission inspections are impending. You are

understandably having a bit of wobbly. The QI light bulb goes of in my head (as the PNA). We together then move into the formative section, I ask some clarifying, explorative and curious questions. One of these questions is have you thought of unpicking your work problems utilising QI methodologies such as a stinky fish? The five whys? We move from the formative into the personal action for quality improvement section. Here is where I ask my final question. What do you want to change? By getting supervisees to write down all their change ideas. Not only are you making the starts of a Driver diagram. You are getting them to switch into deep reflection mode. Which means they are improving their problem-solving and resilience.

To link this back to the asthma clinic example, you can see from the diagram below. Starting from the change ideas the supervisee as then themed the change ideas together. I as the PNA asked how they were going to drive forward those changes' ideas. This then gives us the secondary drivers. I then ask the supervisee how they are going to drive forward the secondary drivers, and this now gives us our primary drivers. Once primary drivers have been thought of, we then conclude with the smart aim of 'Reduce the number of patients missing their asthma check-up appointments at Clinic A by 30% by 31 December 2025.'

The Drivers and the Hinders

Alderwick et al. (2017) define these as things that will be barriers and enhancers to your QI work explored here.

Another common methodology for running a QI project or supporting a QI project is understanding the driver and hindering factors. The driver and hindering factors are quite simple. What is going to drive your project forward and help you to do so?

For example, having the support of your line manager will help drive your project forward. Understanding the issue through the eyes of your line manager ensures joint understanding of the issue.

There is also understanding of what is going to hinder your project – things that will get in the way of your project, such as time and capacity constraints or not having funding. Understanding both is crucial, as it allows the project lead to set realistic expectations for themselves and their stakeholders from the beginning (BMJ 2023). There is never any time or any money to do much, so think realistically what can be achieved with what you currently have at your disposal. My biggest hinder is that I don't have sign off from my manager to do much. So, I get inventive and make it up as I go along. Truly, I invent what I think I can do, and I test it if it works great. If it doesn't work fine, I will learn from the failure and embrace it as my new best friend. Also, finding allies who can help and support you along your journey will be of great help.

Another way of thinking of this concept is to think of a driving bus and a big boulder. A driving bus will take your project from the start to finish. But having a boulder in the way will make the project harder to complete, and you might have to go round the boulder to succeed. Identifying these items or things within your project at an early stage is important. I would advise that the beginning of any project mapping out is not only your stakeholders and how you're going to communicate with them but also your drivers and your hinders.

4. **Who is going to help you change it?**

QI is everyone's responsibility, don't do it alone. The most sustainable projects are those with a team of helpers. Help can come in many forms, such as colleagues, managers and people in different specialities, both internal and external to the organisation where you work.

A project team is also needed; identifying your team early on will help the progression of the project. In the QI world, this team is made of people we refer to as stakeholders, such as senior management, practice development, human resource staff and patients with lived experience. Here is where you need to have a stakeholder matrix (map).

Lining up all the individual stakeholders and then charting them with where they are currently and where you want them to be.

Utilising these tools provides a comprehensive view of what you need to do next and how you are going to bring people along on your journey, for example, stakeholder engagement is like being a train on its journey from London to Glasgow. There are lots of stops along the way, and stakeholders will get on and off at various stations. Stakeholders might love your project but not have 100% of their working time to dedicate to it. They might jump on and off at various points, that's life working in complex systems. It's ok. To mitigate this, having a communication plan with your team and stakeholders is important. It may be a monthly email/newsletter or posts on social media. Updating everyone where you are and what has happened and what needs to happen and from who is important.

5. **How will you know when your change has been successful?**
   Having measures to measure the impact of your project is very important.

   Let's go back to the example of 'Reduce the number of patients missing their asthma check-up appointments at Clinic A by 30% by 31 December 2025.'

   There are three types of measures in QI (state here first and then describe, thanks)

   1. Outcome measure = (achieved goal). This is the measure that shows if your smart aim has been achieved and reflects the projects' goal, i.e. 30% of reducing the number of patients missing their asthma check-up appointments, i.e. more patients stop not attending asthma clinic appointments. Upward trends seen. Brilliant project is working. If the reverse is happening, this gives you as a project team time to stop and relook at the project cycle.

   2. Process measure = (checking if achieving goal). This demonstrates if you're heading in the right direction with your current process in your project.

   3. Balancing measure = (unintended outcomes). These are changes having an impact on another area, i.e. staff are now all burnout in the medical division due to extra audit and documentation.

   Spread and sustainability are also ways we can see success. Other divisions think increasing handwashing should be rolled out in surgical and oncology and they ask you to present how you did this. Brag boldly!

6. **And does it need to be successful?**
   No, is the simple answer. Starting, with a vision of increasing handwashing compliance by 40% is great. But you might not succeed, and you may only get compliance up to 25%. You have still implemented change! Utilising QI methodology, you have still learnt valuable lessons. Perhaps staff need further training around how to wash their hands. Perhaps from doing this QI project, you have identified the problem and can then try to fix it.

   Failure in QI and professional nurse advocacy is not a bad thing. Failure is a good thing because we can learn from it.

In the learning from a failure space, we are reflecting on what went well, what didn't go so well by reviewing, what we could do better next time and what we can avoid.

Future learning is shaped and makes us more resilient not only in QI project management but also in leadership and professional nurse advocacy.

Continuous monitoring and evaluation are key to QI project management.

Setting evaluation milestones through a project is highly recommended. In these milestones, one of the many methodologies I enjoy is 'POKE YOKE' (Shingo 1986), which is a Japanese phrase for avoiding mistakes. It involves trial and test phases to make sure the project is free from error. For example, my project is to carry water in a large bucket. In phase 1 of my test, I place water in the bucket and carry it to the next room. On the way, I notice that water is leaking out of the bucket due to there being holes in the bucket. Before phase 2, I used POKE YOKE (mistake proofing), and this time used a bucket with no holes, and I successfully managed.

Tips for Supporting Others to Run a QI Project

1. As PNAs, we know it isn't our place to give people the answers but to create space for others to reflect.

    This is also true when supporting others to undertake QI.

    We aren't there to give people the <u>answers</u>. We are there for people to run ideas past us and to gently guide the practitioner undertaking the QI project. We suggest not advising.

    This can be incredibly difficult particularly when we have the answer on the tip of our tongue. Important to remember that if we give people the answers, they aren't going to learn or grow. Often going through the motions and making mistakes is the most powerful of lessons.

2. Remember, it is <u>ok not to know everything</u>. QI may be a very new concept to you. Give yourself a break and phone a friend or someone who feels confident with QI. We are all here to learn and develop.

    As I said earlier, not everything has to be QI. Increasing compliance in a hand-washing audit arguably doesn't need to be. This could be a just do project.

    Not everything is appropriate nor will fit into a QI project such as world peace (it's too complex). That is ok too. But QI methodology could be applied, i.e. getting someone through work-related stress. A Driver diagram with the snakes and ladders model could help people you support with next steps and focus their attention to light at the end of the tunnel.

3. <u>Have no fear</u>, be fearless when it comes to QI.

It can be overwhelming at first, and there is an incredible amount to learn.

It can however be learnt. Think back to when you first became a professional advocate you don't know what you don't know.

4. Remember to <u>have fun</u> with this. It's creative and exciting.

Personal Reflection

Working as a professional advocate in complex environments requires persistence, nerve, adaptability and resilience.

Lots of leaders I speak to can't understand me saying how amazing something is and why we should invest in it. But, they do hear and understand me when I show them my measurements for success. A great example of this is no one in the beginning of my journey as a professional advocate wanted to invite me to meetings. Once I started bragging about my measures for success, I suddenly found people were inviting me to meetings. I bragged boldly about a post-evaluation data that asked staff who had come and got support from me. 'How much has the support you received today from Martin, improved your retention in your current role?' 97.5% of the 70 staff I had helped reported that. So, I stopped asking to be invited and I measured what I was doing and then started bragging to people in corridors, who then in turn told others and it kept spreading. Then I became very busy presenting at every meeting I was invited to. What I have learnt is sometimes it starts with a little whisper you may want it to be a loud roar, but don't get ahead of yourselves. It might start with a small whisper than turns into a road. But we start from where we start from and that's ok.

CONCLUSION

Throughout this chapter, we have explored the powerful connection between professional nurse advocacy and QI, recognising that both share a common goal: driving meaningful and restorative change to enhance outcomes for patients, individual staff and teams. By understanding core QI principles and some fun and creative ways, we as professional advocates can utilise these. It really has changed my leadership and improved my confidence to undertake projects. I utilise some of these methodologies not just for QI, but within my practice as a nurse daily and personally with friends. The stinky fish model is one of my favourites to self-reflect on problems I may be having and why am I stuck where I am. It really helps get you out of your head. We as nurses should all be practising reflectively. This helps support our growth and improves our practice. We should be continually doing this as well as part of our revalidation. I have found that using QI methodology has helped my growth as a leader and improved my ability as a nurse, as these tools have supported me to do deep reflection (Moon 2004). 'Deep reflection is a metacognitive, dialogic, and interpretive process where the individual intentionally stands back from an experience to critically explore emotions, assumptions, alternative perspectives, and how their own thought processes shape understanding and learning'. It is not only a profound new tool for problem-solving but also helps with our nursing and midwifery reflective practice, supports revalidation and is a valuable reflective practice we actively encourage among those we support, to foster their growth within QI, RCS or CC.

Even without official power, you can utilise QI tools and methodologies to build engagement, drive conversations, changes cultures and create momentum for change. By applying these principles, you move beyond just seeing problems to actively shaping solutions – transforming challenges into opportunities for sustainable improvement.

My finals thoughts are remembering if I can do it, you can to. Do not compare yourselves to others in anyway particularly in the QI space. As a wise person said, comparison to others is the death of all joy.

There will always be a bigger fish in life and QI, just give it a go, make lots of mistakes, learn from those mistakes and try, try, try again. That really is what I have done.

We work and learn differently. We must embrace our difference as a superpower and all will be well. I wish you well on your journeys and look forward to reading your published QI works. Good luck to you all future agents of change!

REFERENCES

Alderwick, H., Charles, A., Jones, B., and Warburton, W. (2017). *Making the case for quality improvement: lessons for NHS boards and leaders.* London: The King's Fund (and The Health Foundation).

Institute for Healthcare Improvement (IHI). (1990) Science of improvement: establishing measures. IHI Website. https://www.ihi.org/ (accessed 28 December 2025).

Langley, G.J., Moen, R., Nolan, K.M. et al. (2009). *The Improvement Guide: A Practical Approach to Enhancing Organizational Performance*, 2e. San Francisco, CA: Jossey-Bass.

Lees-Deutsch, L., Kneafsey, R., and Wilde, L. (2025). *A Toolkit for Professional Nurse Advocates Undertaking Quality Improvement Work.* Coventry University https://doi.org/10.18552/CHC/2025/0004.

Moon, J.A. (2004). *A Handbook of Reflective and Experiential Learning: Theory and Practice.* London: Psychology Press.

Serrat, O. (2009). *The Five Whys Technique.* Asian Development Bank. https://www.adb.org/publications/five-whys-technique (accessed 28 December 2025).

Shingo, S. (1986). *Zero Quality Control: Source Inspection and the Poka-Yoke System,* (original Routledge edition).e. Taylor & Francis.

Southern New Hampshire University. (2024).

CHAPTER 7

Communities of Practice to Support Well-being

Laura Wilde[1] and Bethany Hall[2]

[1]School of Life Course & Population Sciences, Faculty of Life Sciences & Medicine, King's College London, London, UK
[2]Centre for Healthcare and Communities, Coventry University, Coventry, UK

INTRODUCTION

In the ever-evolving landscape of health care, nurses and midwives are continually navigating challenges, from increasing patient complexity to workforce shortages and emotional fatigue. In such demanding environments, the need for connection, shared learning and mutual support has never been more vital. Communities of Practice (CoPs) provide a platform for collaborative learning, support and innovation, enabling healthcare professionals to share knowledge and improve patient care.

This chapter explores the theory and practice of CoPs in nursing and midwifery. Through real-world examples, practical guidance, and reflective insights, we show how CoPs can enhance professional development, improve patient care and support well-being. Whether you are looking to join an existing CoP or start your own, this chapter will provide the tools and inspiration to get started.

Follow along with the lightbulb 💡 for useful tips on how to put this theory into practice.

WHAT IS A COMMUNITY OF PRACTICE (COP)?

A Community of Practice (CoP) is a group of people who share a common interest or challenge and come together regularly to learn from each other and improve their skills.

> *Communities of practice are groups of people who share a concern or a passion for something they do and learn how to do it better as they interact regularly*
>
> (Wenger-Trayner and Wenger-Trayner 2022).

CoPs can develop organically or intentionally to foster learning, support and collaboration.

In Etienne Wenger's (1998) theory, the core elements of a CoP are:

- **Domain**: A shared area of expertise that defines the identity of the community (e.g. care of the mother and baby for midwives or patient advocacy for nurses).
- **Community**: The social fabric that supports learning and collaboration engaging in joint activities or discussions to help each other and share information.
- **Practice**: The collective body of knowledge, experiences and resources that members contribute to and benefit from as a way of addressing problems.

EXAMPLES OF COMMUNITIES OF PRACTICE

1. **Implementing the Advocate Role into Practice (NHS England, n.d.)**
   The Professional Nursing or Midwifery Advocate (PNA/PMA) role is designed to facilitate Restorative Clinical Supervision (RCS), which provides a safe environment for staff to process experiences, reflect constructively, explore options, and build resilience. The aim is to empower individuals to improve their working lives and reduce stress, making continuous improvement an intrinsic part of professional practice. The PNA and PMA community is a group of

nurses and midwives who come together to integrate the PNA and PMA roles into practice. The CoP focuses on providing peer support, sharing best practices, and fostering a collaborative environment to enhance the implementation of the PNA and PMA role. Due to the national nature of the roles, these CoPs function virtually through the NHS Futures platform, regional and national meetings and conferences.

2. **National Community of Practice for Internationally Educated Professional Nurse Advocates (BMJ Evidence-Based Nursing 2023)**

The National CoP for Internationally Educated Professional Nurse Advocates (IEN PNAs) was established in August 2022 as part of the National NHS England PNA programme. This CoP was specifically created to recognise and support internationally educated nurses (IENs) who have taken on the PNA role. The CoP offers a reflective, restorative and safe space for qualified and trainee IEN PNAs allowing members to process their experiences, reflect on their practice and build resilience. By creating a network of clinical support, the CoP helps IEN PNAs connect with peers, share knowledge, and discuss challenges and solutions. The CoP aims to amplify the voices of IEN PNAs, ensuring their perspectives and contributions are recognised and valued within the healthcare system.

I co-founded the National Community of Practice for Internationally Educated Nurse Professional Nurse Advocates with Emma Perry in 2022, with the vision of creating a reflective, restorative, and brave space for both qualified and trainee IEN PNAs. Co-leading this CoP for two years, I've come to deeply value the role of community in fostering professional growth, resilience and wellbeing.

The CoP has evolved into a vibrant platform where members exchange innovative ideas, reflect on shared challenges, celebrate achievements, and perhaps most importantly, amplify the voices of IENs. It is a space where individuals feel seen, valued, and empowered to contribute their full professional and cultural identities to quality improvement (QI) initiatives.

(continued)

(continued)

Leading this group has underscored the importance of psychological safety and the need to embrace diversity of thought in driving meaningful change.

The impact of the CoP has been wide-reaching: from providing RCS for IENs during winter pressures, to enhancing national visibility, and fostering increased confidence among members to lead and engage in QI work. It has been a privilege to witness the personal and professional development of our members and to grow alongside them.

Kevin Fernandez-Mills
Lecturer, Florence Nightingale Faculty of Nursing, Midwifery &
Palliative Care, King's College London
Co-Founder & Co-Lead (2022–2023), National Community of Practice
for Internationally Educated Nurse (IEN) Professional Nurse
Advocates (PNAs)

BENEFITS OF COMMUNITIES OF PRACTICE IN HEALTH CARE

Communities of practice can offer many benefits in health care, particularly for PNA and PMA. A systematic review, published in PLOS ONE in October 2023, on the aims and effectiveness of CoPs in health care includes several studies demonstrating the successful implementation of CoPs in various healthcare settings (Noar et al. 2023). These examples highlight the practical benefits and positive outcomes associated with active participation in CoPs. CoPs link well with the PNA and PMA roles as they can include opportunities for:

1. **Improved Patient Care**

    By facilitating the exchange of best practices and innovative solutions, CoPs contribute to improved patient outcomes. Collaborative problem-solving within CoPs leads to the development of more effective care models. CoPs have been effective in improving clinical outcomes, enhancing interprofessional communication and reducing errors (Kirigia 2020; Noar et al. 2023; White et al. 2008). This links well with the normative function of the Advocating for Education and Quality Improvement (A-EQUIP) model, which highlights themes around quality issues and professional account-ability, ultimately leading to changes and improvements in how care is delivered to patients, improving both safety and quality (Brunero and Stein-Parbury 2008).

2. **Professional Growth and Development**
   CoPs provide a platform to nurses and midwives for continuous learning and professional growth, such as staying updated with the latest clinical guidelines, advancements in health care and developing new skills. PNA and PMA can share knowledge on best practices, discuss challenges using case studies as examples and develop leadership skills. Informal learning through peer support, advice and mentorship within CoPs can be a great way to keep on top of new developments. The formative element of the A-EQUIP model focuses on the education and development of nurses and midwives to support their practice and improve their leadership skills (NHS England 2023). Connections and networks formed through CoPs can be a great opportunity to support this function.

3. **Promoting Reflection and Critical Thinking**
   CoPs can encourage reflective practice, critical thinking and problem-solving. Having a space where nurses and midwives can critically evaluate their own practice, learn from others, and challenge existing norms can be invaluable. This mirrors what is achieved through the restorative function of the A-EQUIP model, which promotes reflection of personal practice (NHS England 2023).

4. **Collaboration and Innovation**
   CoPs can foster collaboration across disciplines and sectors, for example, midwives working with obstetricians or mental health professionals. There are many examples of innovation in healthcare practices that have emerged from CoP discussions, such as new care models or patient-centred interventions.

5. **Emotional Support and Well-being**
   CoPs offer emotional and psychological support to nurses and midwives, helping them cope with the stresses of their work environment. This support network can help to reduce burnout, provide a sense of belonging and shared experience, and improve overall job satisfaction.

   The biggest challenge can sometimes be taking the initial step to reach out to someone to start a CoP or put yourself forward for an opportunity.

It is important to note that many learning and development opportunities associated with CoPs may take time and require the nurse or midwife to network within the community and take opportunities as they arise.

SETTING UP AND SUSTAINING COMMUNITIES OF PRACTICE

Starting a CoP in Nursing or Midwifery

Having clear leadership is important to ensure the success of a CoP. Leadership may look different across CoPs, for example some may have a consistent leader, whilst others may rotate leadership roles to provide people with opportunities to grow and develop. Starting and sustaining a CoP is not an individual job and requires group effort. There are many roles in starting a CoP that can provide new opportunities for members such as chapter leaders who act as a leader for a local group, connecting them with the wider community and mentors who welcome and induct new members to the group (Wenger-Trayner et al. 2023).

💡 Here are some practical tips for starting and sustaining a CoP:

- **Identify a Common Interest**: Choose a specific area of interest relevant to your practice, such as patient safety or maternal health.
- **Engage Stakeholders**: Reach out to colleagues who share this interest and invite them to an initial meeting.
- **Define Goals and Structure**: Collaboratively set clear goals and a structure for your CoP. This might include regular meetings, rotating leadership roles, and specific projects.
- **Utilise Technology**: Use digital tools and online forums to facilitate communication and collaboration, especially for virtual CoPs.
- **Seek Organisational Support**: Secure backing from your organisation to ensure you have the necessary resources and time to participate in CoP activities.

Virtual and In-Person CoPs

There is growing importance of virtual CoPs, especially in the context of global healthcare networks and the rise of digital health. It is important to consider the best ways for people to access your CoP and tools available for managing virtual communities (e.g. online platforms, forums and webinars) and how they complement traditional face-to-face interactions. Virtual CoPs can be facilitated using these online platforms, making it easier for members to connect and collaborate regardless of location.

Managing hybrid interactions (both online and in-person) can be challenging, but it is important to consider how people who may not be able to attend in person can still access the community and meaningfully engage with it. This could include having an online space or platform where people can access notes, share resources or contact information.

Time and Resource Constraints

A lack of time and resources are very common barriers to regular participation in CoPs, understandably nurses and midwives often feel they do not have time to engage with such activities and a lack of employer/institutional support can make it challenging to sustain CoPs.

💡 Strategies for overcoming these barriers can include:

- Integrating CoP meetings into work schedules (e.g. through calendar invites)
- Securing organisational backing or funding
- Integrate the meetings into time that has already been protected, such as team meetings and study days
- Utilise virtual platforms to minimise travel time and time away from the clinical area
- Making sure the benefits and aims of your CoP are clearly articulated

Navigating Hierarchies and Power Dynamics

There can be challenges of managing power imbalances within CoPs, especially when more experienced members dominate discussions. As a leader (and collectively as a group), it can help to set 'terms of engagement' or an 'agreement' between members. To increase engagement with and adherence to these terms, it can be useful to agree on these together, rather than enforce a pre-set selection of rules. These might include:

- Active listening
- Confidentiality
- Participation is voluntary
- Agree to disagree
- Ask for what you need, offer what you can

Creating an inclusive environment where all voices are valued, and all members feel comfortable contributing is important.

Marjadi et al. (2023) highlight 12 top tips for inclusive practice in healthcare, listed below. We have explored how these points might be considered or demonstrated in your work as a PNA or PMA when forming or participating in a CoP.

1. **Beware of Assumptions and Stereotypes:** *Take note of any unconscious bias that you may be holding, especially when joining a new group that may be made up of people from different backgrounds, cultures, and experiences.*

2. **Replace Labels with Appropriate Terminology:** *Be mindful of the language used within the groups, for example asking everyone to state their pronouns when introducing themselves could normalise this behaviour and help people to feel happy to share.*

3. **Use Inclusive Language:** *Instead of using gendered collective terms like 'hey guys', try more inclusive options like 'hi everyone'.*

4. **Ensure Inclusivity in Physical Space:** *If you are holding your CoP in a physical space, rather than online, it is important to ensure all members can access the space: for example, is there a lift or wheelchair access, is the lighting appropriate for those with visual*

impairments or a neurodiversity. It can be useful to attend the space before meetings to set up and ensure it meets everyone's needs.

5. **Use Inclusive Signage:** *The design of your signs needs to consider accessibility and recognition of people with diverse needs. Think about factors such as font size and type, the colours used, depiction of people (ages, ethnicities, abilities, etc.), and the physical location of the signage.*

6. **Ensure Appropriate Communication Methods:** *Ahead of a meeting, ask people for their preferred communication method. By opening this for discussion, people may feel more comfortable asking for what they need. This may include having information sent ahead of time or being printed out.*

7. **Adopt a Strength-based Approach:** *Allocate roles in the group based on what people can offer, rather than focusing on what they can't. Also, you could offer shadowing opportunities to increase skill sets.*

8. **Ensure Inclusivity in Research:** *Whilst your CoP may not be participating in research, you might like to commit to using evidence-based practice to increase inclusivity in the group and its work.*

9. **Expand the Scope of Inclusive Delivery:** *Nurses and midwives working in clinical, patient facing roles or those working part time might find it more difficult to attend CoP meetings. Varying the days and times of the meetings to ensure more people can attend.*

10. **Advocate for Inclusivity:** *Champion inclusivity and speak up when you see exclusionary practices.*

11. **Self-educate on Diversity in All Its Forms:** *Commit to ongoing learning about different cultures, identities and experiences. This might involve attending workshops, reading, and talking to people with lived experience.*

12. **Build Individual and Institutional Commitments:** *Encourage and facilitate participation in inclusive practices among individuals, teams, and across the CoP and at all levels. Make sure that inclusivity is clearly visible throughout the CoP.*

Whilst these suggestions focus on CoPs, you can also use these principles when you are running RCS sessions, holding career conversations or supporting QI projects.

Successful CoPs can encourage collaboration, empathy and shared learning, fostering a space for anti-racism, diversity, and equity within nursing and midwifery.

💡 **What makes a good CoP?**

A good CoP often has a shared interest, shared activities, and a collection of resources for your practice. For example, this may include:

- Regular meetings
- Collaborative projects
- Share resources and learning (there are many ways to make the most of technology, software and apps for this.)
- Social activities for social learning (e.g. through informal coffee catch-ups, group walks).
- Feedback and feedforward opportunities
- Self-organised and self-governed (collaborating to develop a meaningful and engaging group with membership being optional)
- Cross-professional or multidisciplinary

GLOBAL COPS

CoPs can connect different countries, sharing knowledge internationally and driving global healthcare improvements. For example, global nursing and midwifery CoPs have addressed issues like public health, disaster response, and maternal care in low-resource settings. The Nursing Now Challenge (2021), for example, aims to create leadership development opportunities for early career nurses and midwives from around the world. In 2022, the World Health Organisation launched the Nursing and Midwifery Community of Practice, a network for connecting, collaborating and communicating.

CONCLUSION

CoPs are invaluable for PNA and PMA and closely mirror the functions of the A-EQUIP model, offering a platform for continuous learning, collaboration and emotional support. By actively participating in, or creating CoPs, nurses and midwives can enhance their professional development, leadership skills, and personal well-being. As health care continues to evolve, CoPs will play a crucial role in fostering inclusive, compassionate leadership, and professionals' ability to adapt to new challenges. CoPs will continue to evolve in nursing and midwifery, particularly in response to changing healthcare landscapes, digital advancements, and the need for more inclusive, compassionate leadership. Nurses and midwives should seek out or establish CoPs in their professional contexts to reap the long-term benefits of sustained participation.

REFERENCES

BMJ Evidence-Based Nursing (2023). Setting up a national community of practice for internationally educated professional nurse advocates. https://blogs.bmj.com/ebn/2023/07/09/setting-up-a-national-community-of-practice-for-internationally-educated-professional-nurse-advocates/ (accessed 12 March 2025).

Brunero, S. and Stein-Parbury, J. (2008). The effectiveness of clinical supervision in nursing: an evidenced based literature review. *Australian Journal of Advanced Nursing* 25 (3): 86–94.

Holloway A., Thomson A., Stilwell B., Finch H., Irwin K., Crisp N. 'Agents of Change: the story of the Nursing Now Campaign' Nursing Now/Burdett Trust for Nursing, 2021. Available at: https://www.nursingnow.org/wp-content/uploads/2021/05/Nursing-Now-Final-Report-Executive-Summary.pdf

Kirigia, D.C. (2020). Impact of advanced practice nurses and midwives on patients' outcomes: a systematic review. *International Journal of Health Sciences and Research* 10 (6): 1–6. https://ssrn.com/abstract=3658068.

NHS England (2023). Professional nurse advocate A-EQUIP model: a model of clinical supervision for nurses. https://www.england.nhs.uk/long-read/pna-equip-model-a-model-of-clinical-supervision-for-nurses/ (accessed 13 March 2025).

NHS England (n.d.). Implementing the PNA role into practice: a community nurse perspective. https://www.england.nhs.uk/nursingmidwifery/delivering-the-nhs-ltp/professional-nurse-advocate/case-studies/implementing-the-pna-role-into-practice-a-community-nurse-perspective/ (accessed 12 March 2025).

Noar, A.P., Jeffery, H.E., Subbiah Ponniah, H., and Jaffer, U. (2023). The aims and effectiveness of communities of practice in healthcare: a systematic review.

PLoS One 18: e0292343. https://doi.org/10.1371/journal.pone.0292343.

Wenger, E. (1998). *Communities of Practice: Learning, Meaning, and Identity.* Cambridge: Cambridge University Press https://doi.org/10.1017/CBO9780511803932.

Wenger-Trayner, E. and Wenger-Trayner, B. (2022). Introduction to communities of practice: a brief overview of the concept and its uses. https://www.wenger-trayner.com/introduction-to-communities-of-practice/, https://doi.org/10.1017/CBO9780511803932 (accessed 1 March 2025).

Wenger-Trayner, É., Wenger-Trayner, B., Reid, P., and Bruderlein, C. (2023). *Communities of Practice Within and Across Organizations: A Guidebook.* Portugal: Social Learning Lab. ISBN: 978 989 53290 5 2 (downloadable PDF).

White, D., Suter, E., Parboosingh, I.J., and Taylor, E. (2008). Communities of practice: creating opportunities to enhance quality of care and safe practices. *Healthcare Quarterly* 11: 80–84. https://doi.org/10.12927/hcq.2008.19654.

CHAPTER 8

Cultivating Compassion Within Professional Nursing and Midwifery Advocacy

Bethany Hall[1] and Laura Wilde[2]

[1]Centre for Healthcare and Community Transformation, Coventry University, Coventry, West Midlands, UK
[2]School of Life Course & Population Sciences, Faculty of Life Sciences & Medicine, King's College London, London, UK

INTRODUCTION

Compassionate cultures emphasise the importance of creating supportive and nurturing workplace environments that enhance staff well-being and retention (West et al. 2020). **Compassionate leadership** involves guiding others with empathy, promoting self-compassion and fostering a resilient workforce (West 2021). Finally, **self-compassion** encompasses physical, mental, social and moral health (Dodge et al. 2012), highlighting the significance of well-being in managing the emotional demands of healthcare professions.

This chapter aims to provide a comprehensive understanding of how these concepts can be integrated into nursing and midwifery practice to enhance both professional and personal outcomes. Through practical examples, theoretical insights and real-life examples, readers will gain valuable knowledge on fostering compassionate and supportive environments in their professional contexts.

Follow along with the light bulb 💡 for useful tips on how to put this theory into practice.

COMPASSIONATE CULTURES

The health and wellbeing of nurses and midwives are essential to the quality of care they can provide for people and communities, affecting their compassion, professionalism and effectiveness

(West et al. 2020).

At a time of significant financial and operational pressure, with a nursing vacancy rate of over 40,000 (Royal College of Nursing 2023), the National Health Service (NHS) must focus on improving quality while delivering better value care to its patients and retaining its staff. Despite plans such as the NHS Five Year Forward Plan (NHS England 2014) being introduced with a significant focus on quality improvement (QI), waiting times, pending discharges and staff shortages, unfortunately these staff shortages have continued to increase (NHS England 2017). In this difficult climate, sometimes the focus can move to improving output, rather than on resilience and support of the staff involved. It has long since been recognised that providing positive relationships between the organisation and staff member can be highly protective against stress and reduce turnover (Bennett and Durkin 2000). Therefore, in this section, we focus on how instilling a compassionate workplace culture can contribute to improved staff well-being, retention rates and ultimately enhance staff ability to engage in improving outputs. Developing and maintaining compassionate workplace cultures is essential if we want our workplaces to nurture well-being.

In their seminal work, the 'Courage of Compassion,' The Kings Fund (West et al. 2020) identified the ABC framework of nurses and midwives core needs at work. It is stated that all three needs must be met for nurses and midwives to thrive at work. In the introduction of the professional nurse advocate (PNA) role, it was highlighted that PNAs should work together to support a culture of autonomy, belonging and contribution (West et al. 2020). Together, throughout this chapter, we explore how PNAs and professional midwifery advocate (PMAs) can support nurses and midwives in these areas to contribute to compassionate workplace cultures.

AUTONOMY

The need to have control over one's work life and to be able to act consistently with one's values.

Authority, Empowerment and Influence

Nurses and midwives feel empowered at work when they are able to influence decisions about how care is delivered and structured. It is important that mechanisms are available for nursing and midwifery colleagues to shape the culture and processes within their organisations. This may look different, depending on the type of organisation you work in, and which sector.

PNAs and PMAs can work to support colleagues to have confidence and skills to advocate for themselves and act upon innovations and ideas. They can also use their networks to introduce staff members to colleagues that may be able to support with projects.

While maintaining confidentiality as agreed, themes from supervision and forums can be collated and fed back to the senior management team and professional forums on a regular basis. It is important that QI projects being undertaken are shared and stored centrally, so that the organisation can learn from positive change and avoid duplication of projects.

💡 It can be useful to create a 'You said, we did' document so that nurses and midwives can see how their ideas, thoughts and actions are shaping cultures and patient care. You may also like to link with your patient safety lead to feedback QI projects. It is likely that a challenge in one environment will be reflected in another and there could be valuable learning to be shared.

Justice and Fairness

Nurses and midwives may discuss challenges in their supervision meetings relating to the topic of justice and fairness. These challenges may range from inequitable allocation of breaks on shifts, perceptions of unfair access to a professional development opportunity, to an inability to provide the level of care they believe they should or potentially, the experience of discriminatory behaviours. Whatever the injustice may be, it is important to provide a psychologically safe space for the nurse or midwife to discuss their experiences, work through their interpretations and feelings and make a plan to move forwards. Open questions can be particularly useful at times like these.

💡 These are some examples of open questions which can be used in restorative supervision sessions to explore issues related to justice and fairness. Over time you may like to create your own toolkit of open questions. It could be useful to write these down in a notebook to refer back to.

- Who decides what is just/unjust or fair/unfair?
- You have described this situation as unfair/unjust, but what does that word mean for you?
- What would a more just or fair situation look like?
- Are you making any judgements about the situation/other person involved?
- What don't you know about the situation?
- How might you speak up about your feelings/to advocate for others?
- What steps, if any, have you already taken to address this issue?

Work Conditions and Working Schedules

Having suitable working conditions and schedules is important for nurses and midwives to feel valued at work. While there may be limited input that nurses and midwives can have over their working schedules, there are ways that PNAs and PMAs can help to influence this positively.

💡 Whilst not every nurse or midwife will have influence over working schedules, it is important that a PNA or PMA can still support nurses and midwives who are struggling with their working pattern. This could be through highlighting techniques for work–life balance, signposting to wellbeing apps or support in having conversations to request workplace adjustments, flexible working or changes to shift patterns or roles as needed.

BELONGING

The need to be connected to, cared for by and caring for colleagues, and to feel valued, respected and supported.

Teamworking

Being able to engage in multidisciplinary working is important for effective, patient-centred health and social care. In the context of the PNA or PMA role, it may be valuable to offer group supervision sessions for teams from a particular unit, area or staffing group. This can encourage clear communication as a team and can be especially useful to reflect on an episode of care that has been particularly challenging or very effective. Group supervision can also be used to bring other groups together, such as internationally educated staff members, newly qualified staff members or staff who are interested in a particular topic or area. This opens the space for group learning, connection forming and networking. PNAs and PMAs from an organisation might also like to work together to share resources and learning.

It is also a great form of networking to join communities of practice outside of your organisation. These might be national or international communities of practice for your area of nursing or midwifery such as Community, Intensive Care, or Outpatients. However, a useful community of practice might also be based on a specific interest you have, such as QI.

Culture and Leadership

It is important that PNAs and PMAs enable those they are supervising to cultivate a positive culture and leadership style; however, it is equally important that they lead by example. The role is a clinical leadership and advocacy role, and this is demonstrated in four key ways:

- **Emotional Intelligence:** As reflective practitioners, PNAs and PMAs must be both self-aware and open minded. Through understanding their own emotions, they are able to use these skills to support others to do the same.
- **Integrity**: PNAs and PMAs must always work within their capabilities and The Code at all times.

- **Active Listening:** PNAs and PMAs should be able to demonstrate active listening skills in order to support and advocate for their colleagues.
- **Positive Cultures**: Through utilising the ABC framework (West et al. 2020), PNAs and PMAs will be able to support a culture of continuous improvement which in turn will support nurses and midwives to both thrive and innovate.

NHS England (2023)

💡 A number of these leadership qualities are described as 'soft skills' and are not always tangible or easy to learn. It may be useful to think back on a time when you felt truly listened to or supported by a leader. What did they do or demonstrate that made you feel this way?

CONTRIBUTION

The need to experience effectiveness in work and deliver valued outcomes.

Workload

While we may not have much agency as PNAs and PMAs to impact the workload of our colleagues, what we can support them with are the skills to advocate for themselves if they feel that workloads or allocations may impact patient or staff safety. In order to thrive in their roles, nurses and midwives must be able to deliver safe, compassionate care.

Excessive work demands which exceed nurses' and midwives' capacity to deliver safe and effective care can be damaging to their health and well-being. It is important that nurses are offered the opportunity to attend restorative clinical supervision, during their working time. When staffing is short, opportunities to attend supervision are often limited; however, it is at this time that supervision is the most important. The senior leadership team should be aware and supportive of the PNA and PMA roles to ensure that attendance at supervision sessions is prioritised alongside patient care (Lees-Deutsch et al. 2023).

💡 As a PNA or PMA, it might be difficult for staff to attend sessions when staffing is short and they are busy. It can be useful to offer flexible means of supervision such as visiting the ward with a tea trolley, offering alternative locations or virtual sessions to reduce travel time, or during the walk to appointments in the community.

Management and Supervision

The role of a PNA or PMA is to provide supervision using the A-EQUIP model, which is covered in more depth in Chapter 4. However, in addition to providing supervision, it is essential for PNAs and PMAs to receive supervision themselves. It is difficult to provide supervision when you are not first looking after yourself. This supervision may take different forms. It may be with your lead PNA or PMA, group supervision or even external supervision. Accessing this supervision and sharing the benefits can also help to break down the stigma that is sometimes attached to receiving supervision (Masamha et al. 2022) through role modelling. It is our hope that all nurses and midwives have access to supervision. To achieve this, it can be helpful to have protected time written into the clinical supervision policy at your organisation, if possible.

💡 If you don't want to receive supervision from someone within your organisation, you can connect with other PNAs and PMAs through communities of practice and forums to provide each other with peer supervision.

Education, Learning and Development

Education and development (formative) are a key element of the A-EQUIP model. Throughout supervision, opportunities for learning and development should be identified and action plans created to address these areas. It is important that areas that need addressing are reflected back to supervisees to enable them to prioritise and plan further learning. The use of open questions can be useful again here. Questions such as 'what tools do you think you need to improve in this area?' and 'What does success look like, and how do you get there?' can be used to get the conversation started. It can be useful to remind supervisees that learning identified through supervision can inform appraisals, 1:1s and revalidation.

💡 You may like to create connections with the professional development, practice education or organisational development teams within your organisation. This can help with signposting and ensure that you are up to date on available opportunities, along with the processes around them.

CHANGING CULTURE

A survey of leavers from the register carried out by The Nuffield Trust (Palmer and Rolewicz, 2022) identified that 13% of leavers cited workplace culture as one of their top three reasons for leaving. While a change in culture is crucial, it does not happen overnight. However, small steps can make a big difference when they are made with certainty and persistence. The PNA and PMA community has a wonderful opportunity to role model the culture that we hope to see in our workforce.

💡 If you have any fears or concerns over patient or staff safety, it is always important to know how to escalate these issues, who you can ask advice from and where you can signpost your supervisees to.
   Useful contacts to keep in mind are:

- Your freedom to speak up guardian
- Your safeguarding lead
- Your chief nurse
- Your well-being lead
- HR

LASCHINGER'S EMPOWERMENT THEORY

Laschinger's Empowerment Theory (Laschinger et al. 2001) is rooted in the work of Rosabeth Moss Kanter and focuses on the structural and psychological empowerment of employees within an organisation. This theory is particularly relevant in nursing and midwifery, where empowerment can significantly impact job satisfaction, professional development and patient care outcomes. The theory emphasises the importance of structural empowerment in the workplace. It identifies four key dimensions that are essential for creating a supportive and empowering work environment for nurses and midwives:

- **Access to Opportunity:** Opportunities for professional growth, career advancement and skill development.
- **Access to Support:** Availability of guidance, feedback and resources from supervisors and colleagues.
- **Access to Information:** Availability of relevant information needed to perform job duties effectively.
- **Access to Resources:** Availability of necessary resources, such as equipment, supplies and staffing, to perform job duties.

These dimensions are crucial for creating an environment where nurses and midwives feel empowered and supported.

In addition to structural empowerment, Laschinger's theory also emphasises psychological empowerment, which includes four cognitive dimensions:

- **Meaning:** The degree to which work is perceived as meaningful and aligned with personal values.
- **Confidence:** The belief in one's ability to perform job tasks effectively.
- **Autonomy:** The sense of autonomy and control over one's work.
- **Impact:** The perception that one's work makes a difference and contributes to organisational goals (Figure 8.1).

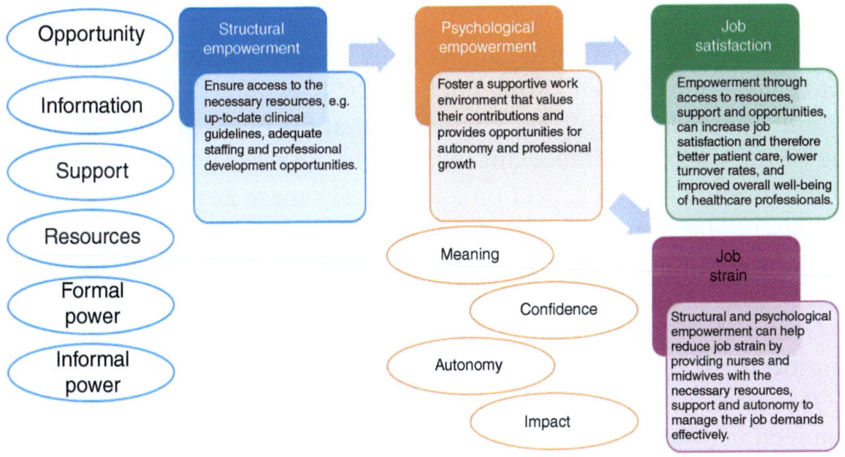

FIGURE 8.1   Laschinger's theory adapted for this chapter. *Source:* Adapted from Laschinger et al. (2001).

COMPASSIONATE LEADERSHIP

While the PNA and PMA programmes aim to equip nurses and midwives with the skills to provide restorative clinical supervision (RCS), support QI and improve safety, their overarching identity is that of a clinical leadership programme. The programme aims to provide those undertaking it with leadership skills to promote and influence positive workplace culture (Sharpe and Hart 2024).

How can compassionate leadership theory be embraced to enhance practice? Throughout this next section, we will explore the four elements of compassionate leadership (Atkins and Parker 2012) that can be used as a vehicle for PNAs and PMAs to contribute to an improved and sustainable workplace culture.

It is recognised throughout the literature that nursing and midwifery staff need to be cared for and supported in order to deliver safe and effective care to their patients (Tierney et al. 2017; Sharpe 2021; Bailey and West 2022). Compassionate care flourishes in a compassionate environment.

In each section, we discuss how each of these elements (Atkins and Parker 2012) can be role modelled and how compassionate leadership can be demonstrated through practice.

ATTENDING – ACTIVELY LISTEN AND HIGHLIGHT KEY CHALLENGES

Active listening is the cornerstone of any PNA or PMAs practice. When active listening is used throughout an RCS session, the PNA or PMA should be able to identify key challenges that the nurse or midwife is facing (West 2021). It is important to facilitate the session in a way that the nurse or midwife can reflect on and identify these key challenges from the discussion themselves. It is not for the PNA or PMA to inform the nurse or midwife of the challenges and how to overcome them, but to guide them through the process of doing this themselves. The PNA or PMA can also help to identify relevant opportunities for innovation and improvement (West 2021), which may lead to additional support through a QI project. Attending in this way can help to nurture a compassionate connection (West 2021).

EMPATHISING – FRAMING 'FAILURES' OR CHALLENGES AS AN OPPORTUNITY FOR LEARNING AND GROWTH

The next element of compassionate leadership is empathising (Atkins and Parker 2012). This has a particular focus on reframing 'failures' as an opportunity for learning and growth. This is a key element of the PNA and PMA role and can be actualised through the 'Personal Action for Quality Improvement' and 'Education and Development' elements of the A-EQUIP model (NHS England 2023). It is important that PNAs and PMAs are able to empathise with a difficult situation the nurse or midwife may have experienced, and again, active listening will be vital. PNAs and PMAs can help the participant identify learning opportunities that could aid them in similar future situations. There may be opportunities to identify QI projects that would contribute to making these challenging situations better in the future or easier for other staff members.

UNDERSTANDING – ENGAGED AND SUPPORTIVE RATHER THAN DIRECTIVE

Linking well with the previous two elements, in order to display compassionate leadership in practice, PNAs and PMAs should be supportive to those they are engaged with, rather than directive. Restorative clinical supervision should not be about having or giving all the answers but about facilitating access to possible tools needed to find answers. This supportive manner enables better engagement and collaboration moving forwards. For example, when a nurse or midwife has an idea for a QI project, the aim should be to guide them through QI methodology, tools to plan, run and evaluate the project and the next steps to take, rather than the PNA or PMA leading on the project. It is important to empower and enable nurses and midwives to do this themselves.

💡 It is important to have a methodological underpinning to the QI work you are supporting. There are lots available and you will likely find a combination that work well for you. There is a national toolkit of QI to support you called 'A Toolkit for Professional Nurse Advocates Undertaking Quality Improvement Work.'

HELPING – REFRAMING, HIGHLIGHTING RESOURCES, REMOVING OBSTACLES OR EMPOWERING NURSES AND MIDWIVES TO DO SO

Intertwined throughout compassionate leadership is 'helping'. There is a fine balance between empowering someone to overcome a challenge themself and removing obstacles to facilitate this process, as opposed to doing it for them. Sometimes the most compassionate approach may not make something easier. It might take you more time to empower and enable someone to overcome a challenge themselves than it would do to take over and fix the problem for them. By being able to highlight resources, reframe challenges and removing obstacles, you will be supporting the nurse or midwife with a new set of skills that they can take with them into the future.

Within my role as a PNA, I started to think how I modelled behaviours of a compassionate leader and did a reflective analysis on my behaviours. I did this both in the context of my team and also colleagues that I would teach and support in practice. I identified that I have created an open culture within my team where people feel safe to challenge and critique me, and each other. This helps us develop our services as well as our own critical thinking, which has had a positive impact on our services. When talking about this with other teams, I try and get them to identify barriers and challenges in creating a similar culture. I often hear that it is due to lack of trust and poor relationships, with historic context that create barriers to people feeling safe to challenge. I ensure that we discuss overcoming this and utilise my PNA skills to facilitate development days that address team dynamics, communication and behaviours in a productive, safe way. Further to this, I identified that I needed to emulate authenticity and be present when I offer supervision. With a busy diary and a busy mind, I would clear both so I could 'attend' and be 'present' to those who I am supervising. I realised very quickly that the impact of this for both myself, and colleagues was much more productive supervision session, and trust building which assisted with honest and productive conversations.

Aimee Hilton, Professional Nurse Advocate.

ANTI-RACISM PRACTICE

In addition to these four elements of compassionate leadership, compassion also implies inclusion and sharing power by encouraging collective leadership (Benevene et al. 2022).

The Anti-Racism in Professional Practice Programme began in 2022 and aims to build consensus on how to promote anti-racism in professional practice (Mello 2023). As a result, the *'Combatting racial discrimination against minority nurses, midwives and nursing associates'* resource was published the following year (NHS England 2022). The resource can be used to provide advice on actions you can take if you witness, experience or hear about racism during supervision. It provides practical examples of how we can challenge racial discrimination. You can also use this resource to empower nurses and midwives to identify and address racism themselves. This is one aspect of leadership where PNAs and PMAs should lead by example, actively ensuring safe working environments, tackling and responding effectively to racial discrimination, harassment and abuse (NHS England 2022).

It is important for PNAs and PMAs to both provide compassionate leadership and practice self-compassion and lead by example – changing the culture over time.

WELL-BEING AND SELF-COMPASSION

Introduction to Well-being and Self-Compassion

In nursing and midwifery, well-being is not a luxury, it is a professional necessity and a foundation for safe, compassionate care. Yet, we know that for many, the idea of 'well-being' can feel distant or even frustrating when basic needs like hydration, rest, or emotional decompression are hard to come by during a shift.

In this section, well-being is examined broadly, encompassing aspects of physical, mental, social and moral health within nursing and midwifery. This section is not about adding more to your plate, but about offering small, realistic strategies that can support your well-being in ways that fit into your existing routines. Self-compassion is not about perfection or unrealistic self-care routines, it's about meeting yourself with the same care and understanding you offer others, especially when things are tough. However, it is important to seek professional support when needed to navigate emotional challenges. This can be done through employee assist programmes, your occupational health department and your general practitioner (GP).

Why Well-being Matters

Well-being is fundamental in healthcare professions, especially in nursing and midwifery, where the demand is both personal and professional. Mental well-being is a key aspect of our overall health, encompassing experiences of happiness, life satisfaction, self-realisation and psychological functioning (Ryan and Deci 2001). Well-being is complex and influenced by many factors. Maintaining our health and well-being involves looking at the resources needed to meet physical, psychological or social challenges (Dodge et al. 2012).

The 2019 National Academies report, *Taking Action Against Clinician Burnout*, defines well-being as an integrative concept reflecting an individual's quality of life, influenced by health, environmental, and psychosocial factors (NASEM 2019). This concept recognises that well-being is about thriving, both at work and in life, allowing individuals to reach their full potential. As humans, we have evolved to develop new types of cognitive competencies, such as reasoning, self-awareness and mindfulness, transforming us into 'super-carers' such as highly trained healthcare professionals (Gilbert 2019).

Challenges to Well-being in Nursing and Midwifery

To meaningfully engage with the principles of self-compassion, we must first recognise the complex and often demanding conditions in nursing and midwifery that shape experiences of well-being.

Common Stressors and Burnout Triggers

Nurses and midwives often face high levels of stress due to heavy patient loads, complex cases and emotional demands. This can lead to anxiety, depression and other mental health concerns, which have been further exacerbated by the COVID-19 pandemic (Getie et al. 2025). Compassion fatigue and burnout are significant risks in nursing and midwifery, often worsened by prolonged exposure to patient suffering and a lack of resources or support (Marshman et al. 2022).

Impact on Mental and Physical Health

The high-stress environment in health care can take a toll on both mental and physical health. Chronic stress can lead to depression and anxiety, as well as physical health problems like exhaustion and reduced immune function (Clarke and Currie 2009). It is essential to address well-being, not just for the individual practitioners but also for the overall functioning of healthcare teams.

Finding a Balance When Returning to Study

For healthcare professionals returning to academic study, finding a balance between work, study and professional commitments can be challenging. The stress and pressure of managing these roles can lead to burnout. It's important to use tools and techniques to maintain a healthy work–life balance and thrive both personally and professionally.

Self-Compassion as a Professional Skill

Self-compassion plays a critical role in promoting resilience, emotional intelligence and maintaining compassion for others in the healthcare field. Just as we advocate for our patients, we must also advocate for ourselves. Even brief moments of self-awareness or kindness can help us stay grounded and resilient in the face of ongoing demands.

Self-compassion involves being kind to ourselves, acknowledging our feelings and emotions and striving to alleviate our own suffering whilst accepting ourselves. Research shows that self-compassion is linked to emotional intelligence, job satisfaction and improved well-being (Nazari et al. 2024). However, being compassionate to others does not always mean we are compassionate to ourselves. Often people find it much easier to be kind and compassionate to others, but neglect their own emotions and feelings, eventually becoming burnt out and exhausted.

Drawing from Compassion-Focused Therapy (Gilbert 2010) and Kristen Neff's (Neff et al. 2020) influential work, self-compassion is described as containing three components:

1. **Self-kindness:** Being gentle with oneself rather than overly self-critical.
2. **Recognition of Common Humanity:** Understanding that suffering and personal failure are part of the shared human experience.
3. **Balanced Awareness**: Maintaining a mindful balance, observing thoughts and feelings without over-identification or avoidance.

Compassion-Focused Therapy (CFT) developed by Paul Gilbert (Gilbert 2010), integrates techniques from **Cognitive Behavioural Therapy (CBT)** with concepts from evolutionary psychology, social psychology, and Buddhist psychology. It focuses on developing self-compassion to manage shame and self-criticism. Key components include compassionate mind training, understanding the three emotion regulation systems (threat, drive, soothing), and developing compassionate inner voices.

Self-compassion enables nurses and midwives to manage their emotional well-being better, which enhances professional quality of life and mitigates burnout and compassion fatigue (Durkin et al. 2016; Beaumont et al. 2016). Notably, whilst being compassionate to others is often a priority in healthcare, self-compassion remains under-recognised.

💡 In your role as a PNA or PMA, you will be supervising and supporting others. It is key to look after yourself, so you can look after others. We do recognise that this can be challenging to do, which is why it is essential to receive supervision yourself as a PNA or PMA.

What Self-Compassion Looks Like in Practice

Self-compassion doesn't require long breaks or perfect conditions. It can be as simple as:

- **Taking a breath** between patients and silently saying, 'I'm doing my best'.
- **Noticing your inner dialogue** and gently challenging harsh self-criticism.
- **Asking for support** when you need it – from a colleague, supervisor or peer network.
- **Letting go of guilt** for not doing everything. You are enough.

- **Positive Self Affirmations** are a powerful practice technique that can help nurses and midwives manage stress, build resilience, and maintain a positive outlook (Pohare and Ganapathy, 2024).
- **Allowing yourself to say 'today was hard'** without judgement and recognising that struggling does not mean failing.
- **Setting boundaries to protect your energy**, even if it means saying 'no' to an extra shift.
- **Offering yourself the same kindness** and patience you'd show a patient, service user or friend.
- **Reminding Yourself**: 'I don't have to be perfect to be worthy of kindness'.

💡 **Example Affirmation Exercises:**

- **Daily Affirmations**: Start your day with positive affirmations that reflect your values and goals. For example, 'I am capable and compassionate', or 'I am committed to providing excellent care'.
- **Gratitude Statements**: 'Today I am grateful that I was able to listen deeply, even though I was tired'.
- **Affirmation Cards**: Create a set of affirmation cards with positive statements. Carry them with you and read them throughout the day to reinforce positive thinking.
- **Journaling**: Write down positive affirmations and reflect on how they align with your actions and experiences. Journaling can help reinforce positive thinking and track your progress.
- **Mindfulness Meditation**: Incorporate positive affirmations into your mindfulness meditation practice. Focus on your breath and repeat affirmations silently to yourself.
- **Visualisation**: Visualise yourself achieving your goals and living according to your values. Use positive affirmations to reinforce this mental imagery.

As a PNA, self-compassion is not just a concept I share with others – it's something I actively practice to remain present, grounded, and effective.

Yoga has become a vital part of this. Through movement and breath, I reconnect with my body, release tension, and create space to reflect.

For me, self-compassion also shows up in quieter ways: allowing myself to pause, acknowledging when I feel overwhelmed, and reminding myself that I, too, deserve care.

Being a nurse and PNA can be emotionally demanding. Holding space for others requires courage. I have learned to recognise my own bravery in this role, and that being kind to myself is not 'a reward' or 'self-indulgence'. It is simply essential.

You spend most of your life inside your own head, best make it a lovely place to be!

Charlee Grace Lystor (she/her), Professional Nurse Advocate.

Small Acts That Support Well-Being

We've framed this section to focus on **realistic, low-effort strategies** that can be adapted to support your physical, emotional, social and spiritual health:

Physical Health

- **Regular Exercise and Movement:** Engage in physical activities that you enjoy, such as walking, running, cycling, swimming or yoga. Stretching at the nurses' station or walking during breaks (when possible) can help release tension.
- **Balanced Diet:** Keep a nourishing snack or water bottle nearby to support energy levels.
- **Adequate Sleep**: Prioritise sleep when off shift. Even short naps or quiet time can support recovery.

Emotional and Mental Health

As well as the self-compassionate techniques suggested above, the strategies below can help maintain and improve your emotional health.

- **Building Self-awareness**: Building self-awareness is the foundation to managing well-being. It enables practitioners to recognise early signs of stress and burnout. Building self-awareness can take time and can be difficult to do at the start. Techniques such as mindfulness, journaling and regular check-ins can help nurses and midwives build a deeper understanding of their personal stressors.

You will likely be familiar with a reflection model already, so making use of this could be really beneficial, for example, reflection models like Gibbs (1998), Kolb (1984) and Rolfe et al. (2001) can be beneficial for self-reflection.

- **Stress Management**: There are lots of stress management techniques and visualisations tools available. It is important to find one that works for you. One example is the stress bucket. This tool helps you to visualise your stressors, unhealthy and healthy coping mechanisms. It can be helpful to draw out your own version of the stress bucket to help identify these in your own life (Figure 8.2).

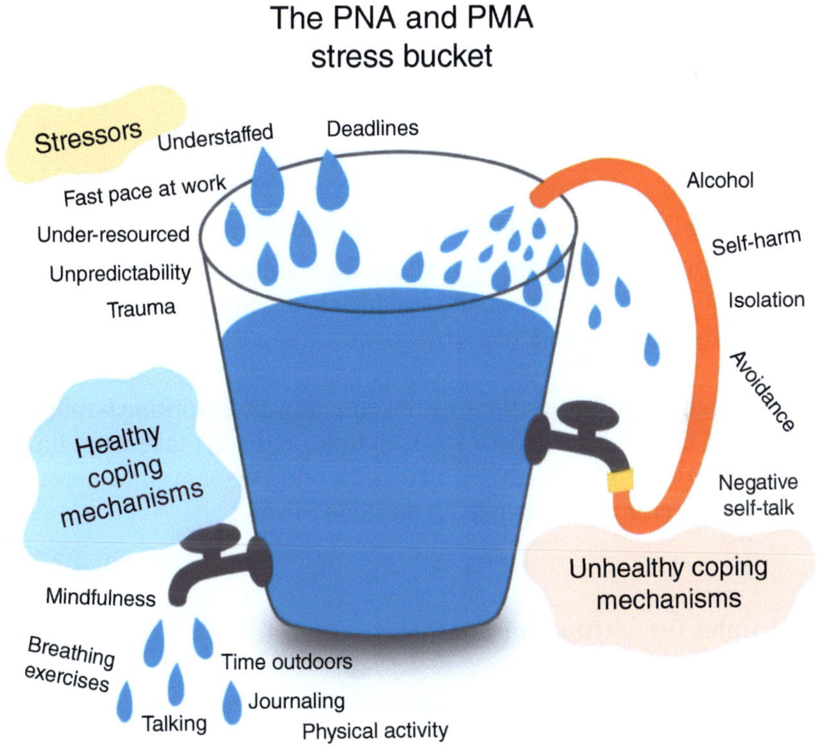

FIGURE 8.2   The professional nursing and midwifery advocate stress bucket adapted for this chapter.

- **Work–life Balance:** Effective work–life balance is a crucial for nurses and midwives well-being. Try to maintain a healthy balance between work and personal life to support mental resilience. Techniques for achieving balance include:
  - **Prioritisation and time management.**

    Using tools like the Eisenhower Matrix and the ABCD method can be helpful to manage tasks effectively.

EISENHOWER MATRIX EXAMPLE.

	Urgent	**Non-urgent**
Important	*Responding to a patient emergency.* **A:** Must do immediately. **Do it** yourself Immediately	*Planning a professional development course.* **B:** Should do soon. **Decide** and schedule tasks to do it later
Non-important	*Scheduling a routine meeting.* **C:** Nice to do if time allows. **Delegate**/automate if possible, do after A	*Browsing social media.* D: Delegate or delete. **Delete,** do not do it, or archive this task

- **Establishing Personal and Work Boundaries**

  Setting clear boundaries is crucial for maintaining balance and preventing burnout, especially for nurses and midwives who may prioritise others' needs over their own.

As a manager, lead by example by not emailing after working hours or on annual leave, ensuring staff leave work on time, and don't take work home.

Techniques include clearly defined work and personal time, especially when working remotely or managing multiple roles.

> ♀ **Examples for Setting Boundaries:**
>
> - **Physical Boundaries**: 'I need personal space, so please knock before entering my room.'

- **Emotional Boundaries**: 'I am not comfortable discussing this topic right now.'
- **Time Boundaries**: 'I am available for work calls between 07:30 and 20:00 on my working days.'

The Nursing and Midwifery Council Code (Nursing and Midwifery Council, 2018) also recommends:

- *To stay objective and always have clear professional boundaries with people in your care (including those who have been in your care in the past), their families and carers (20.6).*
- *To make sure you do not express your personal beliefs (including political, religious or moral beliefs) to people in an inappropriate way (20.7).*

Social Health

Focussing on 'Connection over Perfection' – knowing when to rest and when to connect contributes to your social health.

- **Build Strong Relationships**: Participate in community activities and seek social support.
- **Peer Connection**: A quick check-in with a colleague can be grounding and affirming.

- Join professional organisations or community groups to expand your social network.
- Foster a positive work environment by collaborating and communicating effectively with colleagues.
- Make time for social activities.

Spiritual Well-Being

Spiritual well-being relates to your sense of meaning, purpose and connection to yourself, others, nature or something greater. It is deeply personal and can be nurtured in many simple, meaningful ways. Take some time to consider – what lifts your spirits?

- **Reflect on Values**: Aligning actions with personal values and beliefs can provide a sense of purpose and fulfilment.
- **Micro-moments of Mindfulness**: Use handwashing or walking between wards as a moment to breathe and reset.
- **Nature:** Spending time in nature can be a restorative practice that enhances spiritual health.

> - Take time to reflect on your personal values and how they align with your work.
> - Incorporate mindfulness or meditation practices into your daily routine.
> - Spend time outdoors, whether it's a walk in the park or a hike, to connect with nature.

We understand that time is limited. These strategies are not about perfection; they are about intention. Even small acts of self-kindness can build resilience over time. PNAs and PMAs can play a key role in modelling and supporting these practices, not by prescribing them, but by creating space for reflection, connection and compassion.

A Note on Systemic Support

While individual strategies are helpful, we also recognise that well-being is not solely an individual responsibility. Organisational culture, staffing levels, and leadership support play a critical role. PNAs and PMAs can advocate for protected time, flexible supervision, and compassionate leadership practices that support staff well-being. Returning gently and mindfully to yourself can help identify where systemic support is succeeding and where it needs improvement.

SUMMARY

This chapter discusses the vital role that compassionate cultures and compassionate leadership play in the nursing and midwifery professions. By fostering environments that support continuous learning, collaboration and emotional well-being, these elements contribute to the overall effectiveness and satisfaction of healthcare professionals. This chapter emphasises that compassionate leadership is not only about guiding others with empathy but also about promoting self-compassion among nurses and midwives. As healthcare continues to evolve, the integration of these principles will be crucial in addressing the challenges faced by the profession and ensuring the delivery of high-quality, compassionate care. By embracing compassionate leadership and cultures, nurses and midwives can significantly enhance their professional development, leadership skills, and personal well-being, ultimately benefiting the entire healthcare system. This chapter serves as a practical guide to managing the emotional and practical challenges of a career in healthcare whilst fostering a sense of community and leadership that benefits both the individual and the broader healthcare system.

REFERENCES

Atkins, P. and Parker, S. (2012). Understanding individual compassion in organisations: the role of appraisals and psychological flexibility. *Academy of Management Review* 37 (4): 524–546.

Bailey, S. and West, M., (2022). What is compassionate leadership? The King's Fund. https://www.kingsfund.org.uk/insight-and-analysis/long-reads/what-is-compassionate-leadership (accessed 8 November 2024).

Beaumont, E., Durkin, M., Hollins Martin, C.J., and Carson, J. (2016). Compassion for others, self-compassion, quality of life and mental well-being measures and their association with compassion fatigue and burnout in student midwives: a quantitative survey. *Midwifery* 34: 239–244. https://doi.org/10.1016/j.midw.2015.11.002.

Benevene, P., Buonomo, I., and West, M. (2022). Editorial: compassion and compassionate leadership in the workplace. *Frontiers in Psychology* 13: 1074068. https://doi.org/10.3389/fpsyg.2022.1074068.

Bennett, H.G. and Durkin, M. (2000). The effects of organisational change on employee psychological attachment. An exploratory study. *Journal of Managerial Psychology 15*: 126–146.

Brabban, A. and Turkington, D. (2002). The search for meaning: Detecting congruence between life events, underlying schema and psychotic symptoms. In: *A Casebook of Cognitive Therapy for Psychosis* (ed. A.P. Morrison), 59–75. New York: Brunner-Routledge.

Clarke, D.M. and Currie, K.C. (2009). Depression, anxiety and their relationship with chronic diseases: a review of the epidemiology, risk and treatment evidence. *Medical Journal of Australia* 190: S54–S60. https://doi.org/10.5694/j.1326-5377.2009.tb02471.x.

Dodge, R., Daly, A., Huyton, J., and Sanders, L. (2012). The challenge of defining wellbeing. *International Journal of Wellbeing* 2 (3): 222–235. https://doi.org/10.5502/ijw.v2i3.4.

Durkin, M., Beaumont, E., Hollins Martin, C.J., and Carson, J. (2016). A pilot study exploring the relationship between self-compassion, self-judgement, self-kindness, compassion, professional quality of life and wellbeing among UK community nurses. *Nurse Education Today* 46: 109–114. https://doi.org/10.1016/j.nedt.2016.08.030.

Getie, A., Ayenew, T., Amlak, B.T. et al. (2025). Global prevalence and contributing factors of nurse burnout: an umbrella review of systematic review and meta-analysis. *BMC Nursing* 24: 596. https://doi.org/10.1186/s12912-025-03266-8.

Gibbs, G. (1998). *Learning by Doing: A Guide to Teaching and Learning Methods.* Oxford: Further Education Unit, Oxford Polytechic.

Gilbert, P. (2010). *Compassion Focused Therapy: Distinctive Features*, 1e. Routledge https://doi.org/10.4324/9780203851197.

Gilbert, P. (2019). Psychotherapy for the 21st century: an integrative, evolutionary, contextual, biopsychosocial approach. *Psychology and Psychotherapy: Theory, Research and Practice* 92: 164–189.

Kolb, D. (1984). *Experiential Learning: Experience as the Source of Learning and Development.* Upper Saddle River: Prentice Hall.

Laschinger, H.K.S., Finegan, J., Shamian, J., and Wilk, P.M.A. (2001). Impact of structural and psychological empowerment on job strain in nursing work settings: expanding Kanter's model. *JONA: The Journal of Nursing Administration* 31 (5): 260–272.

Lees-Deutsch, L., Palmer, S., Adegboye, A. et al. (2023). *National Evaluation on Report of the Professional Nurse Advocate Programme: Mixed Methods Study.* ISBN: ISBN- 978-1-84600-1154.

Marshman, C., Hansen, A., and Munro, I. (2022). Compassion fatigue in mental health nurses: a systematic review. *Journal of Psychiatric and Mental Health Nursing* 29 (4): 529–543. https://doi.org/10.1111/jpm.12812.

Masamha, R., Alfred, L., Harris, R. et al. (2022). Barriers to overcoming the barriers: a scoping review exploring 30 years of clinical supervision literature. *Journal of Advanced Nursing* 78 (9): 2678–2692. https://doi.org/10.1111/jan.15283. Epub 2022 May 16. PMID: 35578563; PMCID: PMC9546137.

Mello, M (2023) Anti-Racism in Nursing Practice- Our Duty to Act. The Queen's Nursing Institute of Nursing Practice [online]. Available at: Anti-racism in nursing practice – our professional duty to act – The Queen's Institute of Community Nursing. (accessed 10 August 2025).

National Academies of Sciences, Engineering, and Medicine; National Academy of Medicine; Committee on Systems Approaches to Improve Patient Care by Supporting Clinician Well-Being (2019). *Taking Action Against Clinician Burnout: A Systems Approach to Professional Well-Being.* Washington, DC: National Academies Press (US).

Nazari, A.M., Shahabi, M., Shad, N. et al. (2024). The relationship between self-compassion and burnout in healthcare professionals: a narrative review. *Journal of Nursing Reports in Clinical Practice* 2 (4): 255–262.

Neff, K., Knox, M.C., Long, P., and Gregory, K. (2020). Caring for others without losing yourself: an adaptation of the mindful self-compassion program for healthcare communities. *Journal of Clinical Psychology* 76 (9): 1543–1562. https://doi.org/10.1002/jclp.23007.

NHS England (2014). Five year forward view. https://www.england.nhs.uk/wp-content/uploads/2014/10/5yfv-web.pdf (accessed 10 August 2023).

NHS England (2017). Next steps on the NHS five year forward view. https://www.england.nhs.uk/wp-content/uploads/2017/03/NEXT-STEPS-ON-THE-NHS-FIVE-YEAR-FORWARD-VIEW.pdf (accessed 12 August 2023).

NHS England (2022). Combatting racial discrimination against minority ethnic nurses, midwives and nursing associates. https://www.england.nhs.uk/publication/combatting-racial-discrimination-against-minority-ethnic-nurses-midwives-and-nursing-associates/ (accessed 12 March 2025).

NHS England (2023). Professional nurse advocate A-EQUIP model: a model of clinical supervision for nurses. https://www.england.nhs.uk/long-read/pna-equip-model-a-model-of-clinical-supervision-for-nurses/ (accessed 13 March 2025).

Nursing & Midwifery Council (NMC) (2018) The Code: Professional standards of practice and behaviour for nurses, midwives and nursing associates.[online] Available at: https://www.nmc.org.uk/standards/code/ (Accessed August 10 2025)

Palmer, B. and Rolewicz, L. (2022). Peak leaving? A spotlight on nurse leavers rates in the UK. The Nuffield Trust. https://www.nuffieldtrust.org.uk/resource/peak-leaving-a-spotlight-on-nurse-leaver-rates-in-the-uk (accessed 12 December 2024).

Pohare, A.J. and Ganapathy, M. (2024). Effectiveness of Positive Self-Affirmations on Occupational Stress of nurses in selected hospitals of an urban area. *International Journal of Creative Research Thoughts* 12 (12): 133–148.

Rolfe, G., Freshwater, D., and Jasper, M. (2001). *Critical Reflection in Nursing and The Helping Professions: a User's Guide*. Basingstoke: Palgrave Macmillan.

Royal College of Nursing (2023). Royal College of Nursing responds to the latest NHS England Vacancy Statistics. https://www.rcn.org.uk/news-and-events/Press-Releases/rcn-responds-to-the-latest-nhs-england-vacancy-statistics-aug2023 (accessed 13 March 2025).

Ryan, R.M. and Deci, E.L. (2001). On happiness and human potentials: a review of research on hedonic and eudaimonic well-being. *Annual Review of Psychology* 52 (1): 141–166. https://doi.org/10.1146/annurev.psych.52.1.141.

Sharpe, J. (2021). An exploration of the socialisation of student mental health nurses in compassionate mental health nursing practice: a constructivist enquiry. PhD thesis, De Montfort University. https://dora.dmu.ac.uk/items/526f3aa5-2cc9-4f8a-8faf-5b8e3e401a1d/full (accessed 8 November 2024).

Sharpe, J. and Hart, T. (2024). Applying compassionate leadership to enhance the effectiveness of the PNA. *Nursing Times* 120 (4): 51–55.

Tierney, S., Seers, K., Tutton, E., and Reeve, J. (2017). Enabling the flow of compassionate care: a grounded theory study. *BMC Health Services Research* 17: 174. https://link.springer.com/article/10.1186/s12913-017-2120-8.

West, M.A. (2021). *Compassionate Leadership: Sustaining Wisdom, Humanity and Presence in Health and Social Care*. London: Swirling Leaf Press.

West, M., Bailey, S., and Williams, E. (2020). The courage of compassion. The Kings Fund. https://www.kingsfund.org.uk/insight-and-analysis/reports/courage-compassion-supporting-nurses-midwives (accessed 12 January 2025)

Index